Holiday Harmony

Holiday Harmony

Matthew Petchinsky

Holiday Harmony: A Hydrocephalus Survival Guide for the Festive Season

By: Matthew Petchinsky

Understanding Hydrocephalus: An Overview of Its Symptoms and Impact on Daily Life, Especially During the Holiday Season

Hydrocephalus is a medical condition characterized by an abnormal accumulation of cerebrospinal fluid (CSF) within the ventricles of the brain. This excess fluid causes the ventricles to enlarge, leading to increased pressure inside the skull. Hydrocephalus can occur at any age, though it is most commonly seen in infants and older adults. If left untreated, the pressure on the brain can cause severe neurological damage and even death. However, with modern medical interventions such as shunt systems or endoscopic third ventriculostomy (ETV), many people with hydrocephalus can live relatively normal lives.

What is Hydrocephalus?

The brain constantly produces cerebrospinal fluid, which plays a crucial role in protecting and cushioning the brain and spinal cord, providing nutrients, and removing waste products. Typically, CSF circulates through the brain's ventricles and is absorbed into the bloodstream. However, in hydrocephalus, this process is disrupted, leading to fluid buildup. The condition can arise from a variety of causes, such as congenital malformations, infections like meningitis, brain tumors, head injuries, or complications from surgeries.

Hydrocephalus can be classified into different types, including:

1. **Congenital Hydrocephalus**: Present at birth, often due to genetic factors or developmental issues.
2. **Acquired Hydrocephalus**: Develops later in life, usually as a result of injury, illness, or aging.
3. **Communicating Hydrocephalus**: Occurs when CSF can still flow between the ventricles but is not properly absorbed.
4. **Non-communicating (Obstructive) Hydrocephalus**: Happens when the flow of CSF is blocked within the brain's ventricles.

A unique subtype of hydrocephalus, **Normal Pressure Hydrocephalus (NPH)**, primarily affects older adults. Despite the ventricles being enlarged, the pressure inside the brain remains relatively normal. NPH is often misdiagnosed because its symptoms, such as cognitive decline, difficulty walking, and urinary incontinence, mimic those of other neurodegenerative diseases like Alzheimer's or Parkinson's.

Symptoms of Hydrocephalus

Hydrocephalus presents with a wide range of symptoms depending on the age of onset and severity. In infants, the most noticeable sign is a rapidly growing head, often accompanied by a bulging fontanel (the soft spot on the top of the baby's head), irritability, poor feeding, and vomiting. Older children and adults, on the other hand, may experience different symptoms due to the closed structure of their skulls. Common symptoms include:

- **Headaches**: Often severe, especially in the morning.
- **Nausea and Vomiting**: Associated with increased pressure inside the skull.
- **Visual Disturbances**: Blurred or double vision, or difficulty with eye movements.
- **Balance and Coordination Issues**: Difficulty walking, frequent falls, and poor motor skills.
- **Cognitive and Memory Problems**: Difficulty concentrating, memory lapses, or confusion.
- **Personality and Behavioral Changes**: Increased irritability, lethargy, or depression.
- **Seizures**: In some cases, hydrocephalus can trigger seizures.

For people living with hydrocephalus, these symptoms can vary in intensity and may flare up unpredictably. The condition can be physically and emotionally exhausting, as it often requires frequent medical monitoring and treatment adjustments.

Impact on Daily Life

Living with hydrocephalus can be challenging, as it affects both physical and mental functioning. People with hydrocephalus may face limitations in mobility, difficulty concentrating, and fatigue. This can impact their ability to work, engage in social activities, or carry out daily tasks such as driving, walking, or even maintaining personal hygiene.

In addition to the direct symptoms, hydrocephalus often leads to other complications. The most common treatment for hydrocephalus is the placement of a **shunt**, a device that helps drain excess CSF from the brain to another part of the body, usually the abdomen. Shunts, however, are not without risks. They can malfunction, become infected, or block, necessitating additional surgeries. People with shunts must remain vigilant for signs of failure, which can occur suddenly and require emergency medical attention.

The psychological impact of hydrocephalus should not be overlooked. Coping with a chronic neurological condition can lead to anxiety, depression, or feelings of isolation. Adults with hydrocephalus may worry about their independence, while parents of children with the condition often face stress related to their child's care and development.

Hydrocephalus During the Holiday Season

The holiday season, typically a time for celebration and togetherness, can present additional challenges for individuals with hydrocephalus and their families. The festive period often involves social gatherings, travel, and changes in routine, which can exacerbate symptoms or complicate care.

1. **Travel Concerns**: Whether traveling by air, car, or train, people with hydrocephalus need to be cautious about how changes in pressure (especially with air travel) may affect their condition. Carrying medical documentation, emergency contact information, and ensuring access to nearby medical facilities can alleviate some anxiety associated with travel.

2. **Disruption of Routine**: The holiday season can lead to shifts in routine, including irregular sleep patterns, altered medication schedules, or changes in dietary habits. For individuals with hydrocephalus, maintaining a consistent routine is critical for managing symptoms. Increased stress, lack of sleep, or missing medications can lead to flare-ups of headaches, nausea, or other complications.

3. **Coping with Social Gatherings**: Large, loud family gatherings or holiday parties can be overstimulating and overwhelming for someone with hydrocephalus. Sensory overload, especially in crowded or noisy environments, can intensify symptoms like headaches, fatigue, and irritability. It's important for individuals with hydrocephalus and their loved ones to plan ahead, ensuring quiet spaces for breaks and communicating needs with others to avoid overexertion.

4. **Managing Expectations**: The holidays are often emotionally charged, with expectations of joy and participation in various festivities. For someone dealing with hydrocephalus, balancing personal energy levels and health needs with family or social obligations can be stressful. Setting realistic goals, discussing limitations with family members, and prioritizing well-being over societal expectations are key to enjoying the season while managing the condition.

5. **Support Systems**: Family and friends play a crucial role in supporting individuals with hydrocephalus during the holiday season. Being mindful of their loved one's symptoms and creating a flexible, understanding environment can help reduce the stress of the season. Whether it's providing transportation, adjusting holiday plans to be more accommodating, or simply offering emotional support, a strong support system can make a significant difference.

Conclusion

Hydrocephalus is a complex and life-altering condition that affects many aspects of a person's life. From managing symptoms like headaches, cognitive difficulties, and mobility issues, to navigating the emotional toll it takes, individuals with hydrocephalus often face daily challenges. These challenges can be amplified during the holiday season, a time filled with potential disruptions to routine, increased social obligations, and travel. With careful planning, awareness, and support from loved ones, those living with hydrocephalus can still partake in the joys of the holidays while prioritizing their health and well-being.

Chapter 1: Navigating Holiday Crowds
Tips on Managing Crowded Spaces That Could Increase Stress and Pressure

The holiday season is synonymous with bustling shopping malls, packed public spaces, busy family gatherings, and public events, all of which can be overwhelming for anyone. However, for individuals with hydrocephalus or other conditions that affect cognitive function, mobility, or overall well-being, navigating crowded spaces comes with unique challenges. Crowded environments can amplify symptoms such as headaches, dizziness, fatigue, and anxiety, making it crucial to have strategies in place to manage these situations effectively.

In this chapter, we will explore the impact of holiday crowds on individuals with hydrocephalus and offer practical tips on how to manage these environments to reduce stress, prevent symptom flare-ups, and maintain safety and comfort.

The Challenges of Crowded Spaces for Individuals with Hydrocephalus

Hydrocephalus affects the brain in ways that can make it harder to cope with overstimulation, fast-paced movement, and sensory overload—common experiences in crowded environments. Some of the most pressing challenges include:

1. **Sensory Overload**: Crowded spaces tend to be noisy, visually stimulating, and chaotic. People may be talking loudly, music might be playing, and bright holiday lights may flash around. For individuals with hydrocephalus, who might already struggle with headaches, visual disturbances, and difficulty concentrating, this sensory overload can be overwhelming. It can lead to increased fatigue, confusion, and irritability.

2. **Physical Safety**: Maintaining balance and coordination can be more difficult for individuals with hydrocephalus, making crowded environments a potential safety risk. Being jostled or bumped in a dense crowd could result in falls or injuries, particularly for those who already have mobility issues.

3. **Cognitive and Emotional Strain**: Crowds can also cause cognitive strain, making it hard to process information, navigate spaces, or keep track of personal belongings. The emotional toll of being in such environments can be significant, causing anxiety, panic, or frustration. For people with hydrocephalus, these cognitive and emotional stressors can exacerbate their condition, triggering headaches or other neurological symptoms.

4. **Pressure Changes**: Sudden environmental changes, such as shifts in atmospheric pressure or temperature, can aggravate hydrocephalus symptoms. Overheated malls, enclosed spaces with poor ventilation, or rapidly changing weather conditions as one moves between indoor and outdoor areas can create discomfort or cause an increase in intracranial pressure, which may result in headaches, nausea, or dizziness.

Practical Tips for Navigating Holiday Crowds

Fortunately, with the right preparation and coping strategies, individuals with hydrocephalus can successfully manage the challenges of crowded spaces during the holiday season. Below are some practical tips to help navigate these environments with confidence and minimize the stress and pressure that holiday crowds can bring.

1. Plan Ahead and Choose Optimal Times

Careful planning is essential when dealing with crowds, especially during the holiday season when shopping centers, events, and public transportation are at their busiest.

- **Visit Early or Late**: Whenever possible, plan shopping trips or errands during off-peak hours. Early mornings or late evenings are generally quieter times to visit malls or grocery stores, allowing for a more relaxed environment.
- **Research Events in Advance**: If attending a holiday event is important, research in advance to understand the crowd size, layout, and any accessibility features. Some venues may offer early or exclusive access for individuals with disabilities, which could be a more comfortable option.
- **Create a Detailed Itinerary**: Whether you are shopping or attending events, having a clear plan of action can help reduce stress. Create a list of stores to visit or places to go, and map out the most efficient route to minimize walking and time spent in crowded areas.

2. Use Personal Space Buffers

Maintaining physical space in a crowd is key to preventing accidental bumps or falls, and it can also reduce feelings of overwhelm.

- **Walk with a Companion**: Having someone with you can create a buffer between you and the crowd, making it easier to navigate without the risk of being jostled. A companion can also assist in handling bags, opening doors, or maintaining a steady pace.
- **Utilize Assistive Devices**: If balance or mobility is a concern, using a cane, walker, or mobility scooter can help you navigate more confidently. Not only do these devices provide physical support, but they can also signal to others to give you more space.
- **Strategic Positioning**: When moving through busy areas, try to stay near the edges of the crowd or close to walls where there is less movement. This reduces the risk of being bumped and gives you easier access to exits if needed.

3. Take Regular Breaks

Crowded environments can be physically and mentally exhausting, especially for individuals managing the symptoms of hydrocephalus. Taking frequent breaks to rest, hydrate, and decompress can prevent sensory overload and physical fatigue.

- **Find Quiet Spaces**: Malls, event venues, and public spaces often have quieter areas or seating zones. Plan to take breaks in these areas, where you can sit down, relax, and remove yourself from the noise and activity.
- **Listen to Your Body**: Don't push through fatigue or discomfort. If you start to feel overwhelmed by crowds, headaches, or dizziness, step aside and take a break. Resting for even a few minutes can help you recharge and regain your focus.
- **Carry Water and Snacks**: Staying hydrated and nourished can help maintain your energy levels and prevent fatigue. Be sure to carry water and light snacks, especially if you anticipate long outings.

4. Manage Sensory Overload

Sensory overload can lead to headaches, irritability, and an inability to concentrate, making crowded environments particularly challenging for individuals with hydrocephalus. Here are some strategies to help manage sensory input:

- **Wear Sunglasses or Use Blue Light Filters**: Bright holiday lights and neon store displays can be visually overwhelming. Wearing sunglasses indoors or using blue light filtering glasses can reduce eye strain and prevent headaches.
- **Use Noise-Canceling Headphones**: Noise-canceling headphones or earplugs can help block out the overwhelming sounds of crowds. You can also listen to calming music or white noise to create a sense of peace amidst the chaos.
- **Limit Time in Stimulating Environments**: Avoid spending prolonged periods in overly stimulating environments. It's often better to break up your day into shorter, more manageable activities rather than attempting long outings.

5. Know Your Exits and Emergency Plans

Understanding your surroundings and knowing how to exit a space quickly in case of emergency is vital, especially if you feel unwell or overwhelmed.

- **Locate Exits Upon Arrival**: When entering a crowded venue, take note of the nearest exits. Knowing how to leave quickly can help reduce anxiety and give you peace of mind.
- **Emergency Contacts and Medical Information**: Carry a medical alert card with information about your condition, emergency contacts, and instructions in case of a medical

emergency. This can be crucial if you experience a sudden health issue while in a crowded environment.

6. Manage Stress and Anxiety

Crowds can trigger anxiety for many people, particularly those with hydrocephalus who are dealing with sensory overload, mobility challenges, or cognitive fatigue. Finding ways to manage stress and anxiety in the moment can help keep symptoms under control.

- **Practice Deep Breathing**: Engaging in slow, deep breathing can help calm the nervous system and reduce feelings of panic or stress. Focus on inhaling deeply through your nose and exhaling slowly through your mouth.
- **Visualize Calm Spaces**: If you begin to feel overwhelmed, mentally visualize a calm and peaceful space, such as a quiet beach or a serene forest. This mental exercise can help divert your mind from the stress of the crowd and lower your anxiety levels.

Conclusion

Navigating holiday crowds can be daunting for individuals with hydrocephalus, but with careful planning and self-care strategies, it is possible to reduce the stress and pressure of these environments. By preparing in advance, taking regular breaks, managing sensory input, and staying mindful of your body's signals, you can maintain your comfort and well-being during the holiday season. Additionally, enlisting the help of friends or family members to create a supportive environment can make outings more enjoyable and less taxing. Ultimately, the goal is to find balance, ensuring that holiday activities remain pleasant without compromising your health.

Chapter 2: Understanding Cranial Pressures During the Holidays
How Festive Activities Can Affect Intracranial Pressure and Ways to Manage Them

For individuals with hydrocephalus or other conditions affecting cerebrospinal fluid dynamics, changes in intracranial pressure (ICP) are a constant concern. Intracranial pressure refers to the pressure within the skull, which is determined by the volume of cerebrospinal fluid (CSF), blood, and brain tissue inside the cranial cavity. While ICP naturally fluctuates with activities such as coughing, sneezing, or standing, significant changes in ICP can be particularly dangerous for those with hydrocephalus, leading to headaches, dizziness, nausea, and cognitive impairment.

During the holiday season, the unique combination of festive activities—whether it's travel, changes in weather, or the excitement and stress of social events—can create situations that exacerbate these pressure fluctuations. In this chapter, we will explore how different holiday activities can affect ICP, what symptoms to watch for, and how to effectively manage and prevent dangerous increases in pressure.

The Basics of Intracranial Pressure

Before diving into how holiday activities can influence ICP, it's important to understand how intracranial pressure works in individuals with hydrocephalus. The brain is encased within the skull, and the volume of CSF must remain stable. When this balance is disturbed, whether due to excess production, impaired absorption, or blockage of CSF flow, it can lead to increased pressure on the brain. People with hydrocephalus are particularly vulnerable because the condition already involves disrupted CSF flow, often requiring medical interventions such as shunts to help drain excess fluid.

Increased intracranial pressure can cause a range of symptoms, including:

- **Severe headaches** (often worse in the morning or after lying down)
- **Nausea and vomiting**
- **Blurred or double vision**
- **Balance and coordination issues**
- **Cognitive difficulties** (such as memory problems or confusion)
- **Lethargy or irritability**

These symptoms can be triggered or worsened by various factors, many of which are commonly encountered during the holiday season.

Festive Activities That Can Affect Intracranial Pressure
1. Travel and Altitude Changes
One of the most exciting but potentially problematic aspects of the holiday season is travel, particularly air travel or trips to higher altitudes.

- **Air Travel**: Flying presents a unique challenge for people with hydrocephalus due to changes in cabin pressure during ascent and descent. As the plane ascends, the drop in atmospheric pressure can cause a temporary increase in ICP. For individuals with hydrocephalus, who may already have an elevated baseline pressure, these fluctuations can trigger symptoms like headaches, nausea, or dizziness. Additionally, if a shunt is present, there's a risk that pressure changes might affect its function.
- **Altitude Changes**: Traveling to mountainous regions or higher elevations for winter holidays can also result in an increase in intracranial pressure due to the decreased atmospheric pressure at higher altitudes. The body needs time to adjust to these changes, and for those with hydrocephalus, even mild altitude shifts can lead to discomfort or more serious symptoms.

How to Manage Travel-Related ICP Changes:

- **Consult a Doctor Before Traveling**: If you plan to fly or travel to higher altitudes, it's crucial to consult with your neurologist or neurosurgeon beforehand. They may provide specific guidelines or medications to manage symptoms during the journey.
- **Hydrate Well**: Dehydration can exacerbate ICP changes, especially during air travel, which is notorious for its dry cabin air. Drinking plenty of water before and during flights can help mitigate pressure fluctuations.
- **Move Around During Flights**: If possible, walk up and down the aisle or perform gentle stretching exercises to improve blood flow, which can help regulate pressure within the skull.
- **Adjust Altitude Gradually**: When traveling to higher elevations, try to ascend gradually to give your body time to acclimate. If driving, take breaks along the way to adjust to the increasing altitude. Some individuals may benefit from using supplemental oxygen during high-altitude travel.

2. Cold Weather and Temperature Fluctuations

Winter holidays are often synonymous with colder weather, which can have a surprising impact on intracranial pressure. Cold temperatures cause the blood vessels in the body, including those in the brain, to constrict, which can increase blood pressure and, consequently, intracranial pressure. Furthermore, moving between warm indoor environments and cold outdoor temperatures can create additional stress on the body, potentially triggering symptoms.

How to Manage Temperature-Related ICP Changes:

- **Dress Warmly**: Protect yourself from cold-induced vasoconstriction by dressing warmly when heading outdoors. Wear hats, scarves, and gloves to prevent exposure to extreme cold, which can trigger symptoms.
- **Avoid Rapid Temperature Changes**: If possible, try to limit how often you move between environments with drastically different temperatures. For instance, if you've been outside in the cold, allow yourself to warm up gradually when entering a heated space.
- **Stay Hydrated**: Cold weather can lead to dehydration, especially if indoor heating systems dry out the air. As dehydration can worsen ICP-related symptoms, it's important to drink plenty of fluids throughout the day.

3. Holiday Stress and Excitement

While the holidays are often filled with joy and excitement, they can also bring significant stress, whether from planning events, shopping, or managing family dynamics. Emotional stress has a well-documented effect on physical health, and for individuals with hydrocephalus, stress can trigger an increase in intracranial pressure.

When the body is stressed, it releases hormones like cortisol and adrenaline, which can increase heart rate and blood pressure. For individuals with hydrocephalus, this can cause an unwanted increase in ICP, leading to symptoms like headaches, irritability, and difficulty concentrating.

How to Manage Holiday Stress:

- **Prioritize Self-Care**: One of the best ways to manage stress during the holidays is by making self-care a priority. This can include simple practices such as ensuring you get enough sleep, taking breaks from holiday preparations, and engaging in relaxing activities like meditation or deep breathing exercises.
- **Pace Yourself**: Don't feel pressured to do everything at once. Spread out your activities and tasks over several days to avoid overwhelming yourself. For instance, instead of cramming all your shopping into one day, plan shorter trips over a week or two.
- **Set Boundaries**: While holiday gatherings can be a source of joy, they can also be overwhelming, especially if you're dealing with family dynamics or expectations. Set clear boundaries about what you're comfortable with, whether it's limiting the length of time you spend at events or declining invitations to overly stressful gatherings.

4. Physical Exertion and Overexertion

Many holiday traditions involve physical activities such as decorating, cooking, or playing with children or grandchildren. While moderate physical activity can be beneficial for overall health, overexertion can lead to increased ICP, especially in individuals with hydrocephalus. Straining, heavy lifting, or engaging in intense physical activities can cause sudden spikes in intracranial pressure.

How to Manage Physical Exertion:

- **Take Frequent Breaks**: If you're engaging in physical activities like decorating or cooking, take frequent breaks to avoid overexertion. Listen to your body, and stop if you begin to feel fatigued, dizzy, or experience a headache.
- **Avoid Straining**: Be mindful of activities that involve heavy lifting, bending over, or straining, as these can increase pressure inside the skull. If needed, ask for help with tasks that require more physical effort.
- **Stay Active in Moderation**: While intense physical exertion should be avoided, light to moderate physical activity, such as walking or stretching, can improve circulation and help regulate intracranial pressure. Gentle exercise can also reduce stress, making it an excellent way to stay active during the holidays without triggering symptoms.

5. Dietary Factors and Holiday Foods

Holiday meals and treats are a big part of the festive season, but certain foods and beverages can impact intracranial pressure. High-sodium foods, for example, can cause the body to retain fluid, which may lead to an increase in blood pressure and ICP. Similarly, excessive caffeine or alcohol consumption can dehydrate the body, leading to an increase in ICP symptoms like headaches and nausea.

How to Manage Dietary Triggers:

- **Monitor Sodium Intake**: Be mindful of high-sodium foods, which are common in holiday meals (such as cured meats, processed snacks, and certain soups). Opt for low-sodium alternatives when possible, and balance your meals with plenty of fruits and vegetables.
- **Stay Hydrated**: Drinking plenty of water throughout the day is essential, especially if you're consuming caffeine or alcohol. Staying hydrated can help maintain stable intracranial pressure and prevent dehydration-related headaches.
- **Limit Caffeine and Alcohol**: While it's tempting to enjoy a few extra cups of coffee or indulge in holiday cocktails, it's important to consume these in moderation. Both caffeine and alcohol can contribute to dehydration, which may worsen ICP-related symptoms.

Recognizing Dangerous ICP Symptoms During the Holidays

While holiday activities can create situations that may lead to increased intracranial pressure, it's essential to be aware of the warning signs that indicate more serious problems. Symptoms to watch for include:

- **Persistent or severe headaches** that are not relieved by rest or over-the-counter pain medications
- **Nausea and vomiting**, especially if accompanied by headaches or visual disturbances
- **Sudden vision changes**, such as blurred or double vision
- **Unexplained drowsiness or lethargy**
- **Cognitive difficulties**, such as confusion, memory problems, or difficulty concentrating
- **Balance and coordination issues**, especially if you notice a sudden change in your ability to walk or move

If you experience any of these symptoms, it's important to seek medical attention immediately. Severe ICP increases can be life-threatening if left untreated.

Conclusion

Understanding the relationship between holiday activities and intracranial pressure is key to managing your health during the festive season. Whether you're traveling, participating in physical activities, or enjoying holiday foods, being mindful of how these experiences can impact your condition will help you prevent symptom flare-ups and keep your ICP under control. By prioritizing self-care, managing stress, and recognizing the warning signs of increased pressure, you can enjoy the holidays while maintaining your well-being and safety.

Chapter 3: Recognizing Holiday Stress Triggers
Identifying the Unique Stressors That May Exacerbate Hydrocephalus Symptoms

The holiday season is often a time of joy and celebration, filled with family gatherings, social events, and festive traditions. However, for individuals living with hydrocephalus, the holidays can also bring a unique set of stressors that can exacerbate symptoms and increase intracranial pressure (ICP). Stress has a profound effect on the body and brain, and for those with hydrocephalus, even small changes in routine, environment, or emotional state can trigger symptoms such as headaches, nausea, dizziness, and cognitive difficulties.

Recognizing the specific stress triggers during the holiday season is essential for managing hydrocephalus symptoms effectively. In this chapter, we will explore the various holiday-related stressors that can impact individuals with hydrocephalus, how these stressors can increase ICP, and strategies for managing and minimizing these triggers.

How Stress Affects Hydrocephalus Symptoms

Stress is the body's natural response to challenges or demands, and it activates a complex chain of physiological reactions known as the "fight-or-flight" response. When you experience stress, your body releases hormones such as cortisol and adrenaline, which increase heart rate, blood pressure, and overall alertness. While this response is helpful in short-term, high-pressure situations, chronic stress or repeated exposure to stressful events can have negative consequences—particularly for individuals with hydrocephalus.

For those with hydrocephalus, increased stress can contribute to the following:

1. **Increased Intracranial Pressure (ICP)**: Stress hormones can lead to higher blood pressure, which in turn can raise ICP. Elevated ICP can exacerbate symptoms such as headaches, visual disturbances, and nausea.
2. **Cognitive Fatigue**: Stress can cause mental fatigue and impair cognitive function, making it harder to focus, remember things, or engage in conversations—all of which are already challenges for individuals with hydrocephalus.
3. **Emotional Strain**: Stress can also amplify feelings of anxiety, frustration, or irritability, which can create a vicious cycle of worsening symptoms and emotional distress.
4. **Physical Symptoms**: The body's response to stress can manifest physically as muscle tension, rapid heartbeat, or digestive issues, all of which can further contribute to discomfort for someone managing a chronic condition.

Holiday Stress Triggers That Can Exacerbate Hydrocephalus Symptoms

The holiday season introduces several stressors that are unique to this time of year. These stressors can vary from person to person, but individuals with hydrocephalus may be particularly sensitive to the following triggers:

1. Disruption of Routine

One of the most significant stressors during the holidays is the disruption of daily routines. Regular schedules—including sleep patterns, medication timings, meal times, and rest periods—can become difficult to maintain when social events, travel, and celebrations take precedence.

- **Impact on Hydrocephalus**: People with hydrocephalus often rely on a consistent routine to manage symptoms and maintain their health. A disrupted routine can lead to missed medications, irregular sleep, and inadequate rest, all of which can increase ICP and trigger symptoms.
- **Management Strategies**:
    - **Prioritize Your Routine**: As much as possible, try to maintain regular sleep, meal, and medication schedules, even during the busiest parts of the holiday season. If you have a set time for taking medication or resting, plan your social activities around these critical health priorities.
    - **Communicate with Others**: Don't hesitate to communicate your needs to family and friends. If you need to excuse yourself to take medication or rest during an event, let your hosts know in advance to reduce stress or pressure.

2. Social Obligations and Family Gatherings

The holiday season is often filled with social obligations, from large family gatherings to work parties and community events. While these events can be enjoyable, they can also be overwhelming, particularly for individuals with hydrocephalus who may struggle with sensory overload, fatigue, or cognitive challenges.

- **Impact on Hydrocephalus**: Large gatherings often involve noisy environments, long conversations, and crowded spaces, which can trigger headaches, confusion, or emotional exhaustion. Additionally, the pressure to socialize and meet the expectations of family members can cause significant emotional stress.
- **Management Strategies**:
    - **Set Boundaries**: It's essential to set realistic limits on how much social activity you can manage. If large gatherings or back-to-back events feel overwhelming, choose to attend only a few key events and politely decline others. Don't feel obligated to attend every invitation.

- **Take Breaks**: If you do attend social events, give yourself permission to take breaks. Step outside for some fresh air or find a quiet space to sit and decompress if you begin to feel overwhelmed by the noise and activity.
- **Use Coping Tools**: Consider using tools such as noise-canceling headphones, sunglasses (for bright holiday lights), or visual focus points to help reduce sensory overload.

3. Holiday Shopping and Crowds

Holiday shopping is a stressor for many people, but for individuals with hydrocephalus, navigating crowded malls, stores, or holiday markets can be physically and mentally taxing. The noise, movement, and visual stimulation in crowded environments can quickly lead to fatigue and headaches.

- **Impact on Hydrocephalus**: Crowded spaces can trigger sensory overload, balance issues, or anxiety, all of which can exacerbate hydrocephalus symptoms. The stress of navigating busy stores and long lines can also lead to increased ICP and physical exhaustion.
- **Management Strategies**:
  - **Shop During Off-Peak Hours**: Avoid the busiest shopping times, such as weekends and evenings, by planning shopping trips during quieter hours. Early mornings or weekday afternoons tend to be less crowded and more manageable.
  - **Use Online Shopping**: If in-person shopping feels too overwhelming, take advantage of online shopping options. Many stores offer free shipping or in-store pickup, allowing you to avoid the stress of crowds altogether.
  - **Delegate Tasks**: If possible, delegate shopping tasks to family members or friends. You can also consider buying gift cards or making homemade gifts to simplify the shopping process.

4. Financial Pressures

The holiday season often comes with financial stress, whether it's the pressure to buy gifts, travel to see family, or host large gatherings. Financial worries can trigger significant emotional stress, which may exacerbate hydrocephalus symptoms.

- **Impact on Hydrocephalus**: Financial concerns can lead to anxiety, irritability, and sleeplessness, all of which can worsen ICP-related symptoms like headaches or cognitive difficulties.
- **Management Strategies**:
  - **Set a Budget**: Create a realistic holiday budget that accounts for gifts, travel, and other holiday expenses. Stick to this budget to avoid financial strain and minimize stress.
  - **Simplify Gift-Giving**: Consider simplifying gift-giving by opting for meaningful, low-cost gifts, such as homemade items or experiences rather than expensive presents. You can also suggest a family gift exchange, where each person buys only one gift for a designated family member.

- ◦ **Communicate with Loved Ones**: If finances are a concern, communicate openly with your loved ones about setting realistic expectations for the holidays. Most people will be understanding and supportive.

5. Travel-Related Stress

For many, the holidays involve travel—whether it's flying to visit family, driving long distances, or taking public transportation. Travel can be stressful for anyone, but for individuals with hydrocephalus, it can bring specific challenges, such as managing ICP changes due to altitude or pressure changes, staying comfortable during long journeys, and keeping up with medication schedules.

- **Impact on Hydrocephalus**: Travel-related stress can cause increased ICP, especially if travel involves flying or visiting high-altitude locations. Additionally, the disruption of routine, sleep, and dietary habits during travel can trigger headaches, nausea, and cognitive fatigue.
- **Management Strategies**:
    - ◦ **Plan Ahead**: Make sure to plan your travel in advance, including booking accessible accommodations, mapping out rest stops during long drives, and packing all necessary medications and medical documentation.
    - ◦ **Manage ICP During Flights**: If flying, consult with your doctor beforehand about ways to manage ICP changes. Staying hydrated, moving around the cabin when possible, and using pressure-regulating earplugs can help alleviate symptoms.
    - ◦ **Take Breaks During Road Trips**: For long car trips, plan to take frequent breaks to stretch, move around, and rest. This can help prevent the buildup of ICP from sitting for extended periods.

6. Pressure to Meet Expectations

The holiday season often comes with expectations—from family traditions to social obligations and personal goals for the "perfect" holiday experience. The pressure to meet these expectations, whether imposed by others or self-imposed, can lead to significant emotional stress.

- **Impact on Hydrocephalus**: The pressure to meet holiday expectations can cause anxiety, frustration, and exhaustion, all of which can increase ICP and worsen symptoms. The desire to "keep up" with others or maintain traditional holiday routines can be particularly draining for individuals managing a chronic condition like hydrocephalus.
- **Management Strategies**:
    - ◦ **Adjust Expectations**: Recognize that it's okay to adjust your holiday expectations to suit your current health and energy levels. Let go of the idea of a "perfect" holiday and focus on what brings you joy and comfort.
    - ◦ **Delegate Tasks**: If you're hosting an event or managing holiday preparations, don't be afraid to delegate tasks to others. Whether it's asking a family member to help with cooking or letting someone else take the lead on organizing, sharing responsibilities can significantly reduce stress.

- ° **Practice Self-Compassion**: Be kind to yourself during the holidays. Recognize that managing a chronic condition like hydrocephalus comes with limitations, and it's okay to prioritize your well-being over societal or family expectations.

Conclusion

The holiday season is filled with opportunities for joy and connection, but it can also be a time of heightened stress, especially for individuals with hydrocephalus. Recognizing the unique stressors that may arise—whether from disrupted routines, social obligations, financial pressures, or travel—is the first step in managing and minimizing their impact on your health. By setting realistic boundaries, planning ahead, and prioritizing self-care, you can reduce the risk of exacerbating hydrocephalus symptoms and create a holiday experience that is enjoyable, manageable, and supportive of your well-being.

Chapter 4: Temperature Fluctuations and Cranial Pressure
Managing Cranial Pressure During Sudden Changes in Temperature, Particularly During Winter

For individuals with hydrocephalus or other conditions that affect intracranial pressure (ICP), changes in temperature—especially sudden fluctuations—can have a significant impact on their symptoms. The winter season presents a unique set of challenges, as cold weather, wind chill, and transitions between indoor and outdoor environments can trigger discomfort and lead to an increase in intracranial pressure. Understanding how temperature affects the body and brain, and learning how to manage these fluctuations, is essential for maintaining comfort and well-being during the winter months.

In this chapter, we will explore how sudden changes in temperature affect cranial pressure, the symptoms that may arise in cold weather, and practical strategies for managing these fluctuations effectively.

Understanding Temperature and Intracranial Pressure

Intracranial pressure is the pressure exerted by the cerebrospinal fluid (CSF) inside the skull. For individuals with hydrocephalus, the normal flow and absorption of CSF are disrupted, often leading to elevated pressure inside the skull. ICP can fluctuate based on various external and internal factors, including physical activity, body position, stress levels, and environmental conditions—particularly temperature.

Temperature fluctuations affect the body in several ways, which can directly or indirectly influence ICP:

1. **Vasoconstriction and Vasodilation**: Exposure to cold temperatures causes the blood vessels in the body, including those in the brain, to constrict (vasoconstriction). This physiological response helps preserve core body heat but can also increase blood pressure, which may lead to higher ICP. Conversely, moving from a cold environment to a warm one can cause the blood vessels to dilate (vasodilation), resulting in rapid shifts in blood flow that may further impact ICP.

2. **Thermal Stress**: Rapid changes in temperature, such as moving from a warm indoor environment to a cold outdoor setting, can create stress on the body. Thermal stress occurs when the body struggles to maintain its normal temperature, triggering responses that can increase blood pressure and ICP. This is especially problematic for individuals with hydrocephalus, as their ability to regulate ICP may already be compromised.

3. **Shivering and Muscle Tension**: In cold environments, the body reacts by shivering to generate heat and by tightening muscles to conserve warmth. These physical responses can lead to increased muscle tension and a rise in intracranial pressure due to changes in overall blood flow and oxygen consumption.

4. **Dehydration**: Cold weather can also lead to dehydration, as people may not feel as thirsty in the winter as they do in warmer months. Dehydration can cause the body to retain fluids, potentially leading to increased ICP and other symptoms.

Symptoms of Temperature-Related ICP Changes

For individuals with hydrocephalus, temperature fluctuations can cause a range of symptoms, particularly if ICP rises in response to cold or sudden temperature changes. Some common symptoms that may be experienced during cold weather or abrupt shifts between indoor and outdoor environments include:

- **Headaches**: One of the most common symptoms of increased ICP is headaches, which may become more intense in cold weather or when transitioning between environments.
- **Nausea and Vomiting**: Sudden shifts in ICP can trigger nausea and, in severe cases, vomiting. This is especially common in cold environments, where the body's reaction to temperature stress may cause a spike in pressure.
- **Visual Disturbances**: Changes in ICP can affect vision, leading to symptoms like blurred or double vision, which may worsen during temperature fluctuations.
- **Dizziness and Balance Issues**: The cold weather can also exacerbate dizziness or problems with balance, especially if ICP increases.
- **Fatigue and Cognitive Difficulties**: Sudden changes in cranial pressure can cause fatigue, confusion, and difficulty concentrating, as the brain struggles to cope with the shifts in blood flow and oxygen supply.

Managing Cranial Pressure During Cold Weather and Temperature Fluctuations

While it is impossible to completely avoid temperature changes during the winter, there are several strategies that individuals with hydrocephalus can use to manage their symptoms and minimize the impact of temperature fluctuations on cranial pressure. These strategies focus on maintaining a stable body temperature, reducing thermal stress, and preventing triggers that could lead to an increase in ICP.

1. Dress in Layers to Regulate Body Temperature

One of the most effective ways to manage temperature fluctuations is to dress in layers. Layering allows you to easily add or remove clothing as needed, helping you maintain a consistent body temperature as you transition between indoor and outdoor environments.

- **Wear a Hat and Scarf**: Heat loss occurs most rapidly through the head, so wearing a hat or scarf is crucial for retaining warmth. Opt for breathable, insulating fabrics such as wool or fleece, which provide warmth without causing overheating.
- **Layer Your Clothing**: Choose multiple layers of clothing, such as a base layer made of moisture-wicking fabric to keep sweat away from your skin, a mid-layer for insulation (like fleece or down), and an outer layer that protects against wind and moisture. This approach allows you to adjust your clothing as temperatures change.

- **Keep Extremities Warm**: Cold hands and feet can trigger the body's overall response to cold, leading to vasoconstriction and an increase in ICP. Wear gloves and warm socks to ensure your extremities are well-protected.

2. Limit Time Spent in Extreme Cold

Prolonged exposure to very cold temperatures can increase the risk of ICP-related symptoms, so it's important to limit your time outdoors in extreme cold and take steps to warm up when necessary.

- **Take Breaks Indoors**: If you need to be outside for an extended period, take breaks indoors to warm up and allow your body to recover from the cold.
- **Avoid Extreme Temperatures**: Try to avoid being outside during the coldest parts of the day, typically early in the morning or late at night. If possible, schedule outdoor activities during warmer periods of the day when the sun is shining.
- **Use Heating Pads or Warmers**: Portable heating pads or hand warmers can be useful for keeping your body warm without the need for heavy physical exertion, which could raise ICP.

3. Manage Transitions Between Indoor and Outdoor Environments

Rapid transitions between the cold outdoors and warm indoor environments can create thermal stress, which may increase ICP and trigger symptoms such as headaches or nausea. It's important to manage these transitions carefully to avoid sudden shifts in body temperature.

- **Allow Time to Acclimate**: When transitioning from the cold outdoors to a warm indoor environment (or vice versa), give your body time to acclimate. Stay near the entrance for a few moments to let your body adjust gradually to the temperature change.
- **Avoid Overheating Indoors**: While it's important to stay warm indoors, overheating can also be problematic, leading to dehydration or increased blood flow to the brain, which can raise ICP. Keep indoor temperatures at a comfortable, moderate level and avoid sitting too close to direct heat sources like radiators or fireplaces.
- **Hydrate After Temperature Shifts**: Make sure to drink water after transitioning between cold and warm environments to maintain hydration and reduce the risk of dehydration-related ICP increases.

4. Stay Hydrated

Dehydration can worsen symptoms of increased ICP, and during the winter months, it's easy to become dehydrated without realizing it. Cold weather often suppresses the sensation of thirst, so people tend to drink less water in the winter than in warmer months. Additionally, indoor heating systems can create dry air, leading to fluid loss through the skin and respiratory system.

- **Drink Water Regularly**: Even if you don't feel thirsty, make a conscious effort to drink water throughout the day. Keeping a water bottle with you can serve as a reminder to stay hydrated.
- **Monitor Urine Color**: A good indicator of hydration levels is the color of your urine—if it's dark yellow, it's a sign that you need to drink more water. Clear or light yellow urine indicates proper hydration.
- **Limit Caffeine and Alcohol**: Both caffeine and alcohol can lead to dehydration, which can exacerbate ICP-related symptoms. Be mindful of your intake, especially during social events or gatherings.

5. Avoid Overexertion in Cold Weather

While staying physically active is important for overall health, overexertion in cold weather can lead to increased ICP. The body works harder to stay warm in the cold, and intense physical activity can cause a spike in blood pressure and ICP, which may trigger headaches, dizziness, or nausea.

- **Take It Slow**: Avoid strenuous outdoor activities such as shoveling snow, jogging in the cold, or heavy lifting, especially in very cold temperatures. Opt for lighter activities, such as walking, that are less likely to increase ICP.
- **Warm Up Gradually**: If you're planning to engage in outdoor activities, take time to warm up gradually by doing light stretching or indoor exercises before heading outside. This can help prevent sudden spikes in blood pressure.
- **Listen to Your Body**: Pay attention to how your body feels during cold-weather activities. If you start to feel fatigued, dizzy, or experience a headache, stop and rest immediately.

6. Recognize Warning Signs of Increased ICP

It's important to be aware of the warning signs that indicate your intracranial pressure may be rising in response to temperature changes. Knowing these symptoms can help you take action before they become severe.

- **Headaches**: Persistent or worsening headaches are one of the primary signs of increased ICP. If you notice that your headaches intensify in cold weather or after sudden temperature changes, take steps to warm up and rest.

- **Nausea and Dizziness**: If you experience nausea or dizziness, especially after moving between cold and warm environments, it could be a sign that your ICP is fluctuating. Rest in a warm, comfortable environment and drink water to help stabilize your body.
- **Visual Disturbances**: Blurred or double vision may indicate that your ICP has risen. If this occurs, seek medical attention if symptoms persist or worsen.

Conclusion

Temperature fluctuations during the winter months can have a significant impact on individuals with hydrocephalus, particularly when it comes to managing intracranial pressure. Cold weather, rapid shifts between indoor and outdoor environments, and physical exertion can all lead to changes in ICP, triggering symptoms such as headaches, dizziness, and nausea. By understanding how temperature affects cranial pressure and implementing strategies to manage these fluctuations—such as dressing in layers, staying hydrated, limiting exposure to extreme cold, and avoiding overexertion—you can reduce the risk of symptom flare-ups and maintain comfort during the winter season.

Staying mindful of your body's responses to temperature changes, planning ahead, and practicing self-care will help ensure that you can enjoy the winter holidays and colder months while keeping your cranial pressure under control.

Chapter 5: Wearing Winter Gear Comfortably
How to Choose Hats and Scarves That Won't Put Pressure on the Head or Shunt

Winter gear—particularly hats and scarves—is essential for staying warm and protecting yourself from the cold, especially during the winter months. However, for individuals with hydrocephalus or those who have a shunt placed to manage intracranial pressure (ICP), wearing winter accessories can present unique challenges. The head, which is a key area for regulating body heat, can be sensitive to external pressure. A poorly fitted hat or scarf can cause discomfort, headaches, or even interfere with the function of a shunt, which is typically located in the head or neck.

This chapter will provide detailed guidance on selecting and wearing winter hats and scarves in a way that ensures warmth and comfort without putting unnecessary pressure on the head or compromising the function of a shunt.

Understanding the Importance of Proper Winter Gear for Individuals with Hydrocephalus

For individuals with hydrocephalus, temperature regulation and cranial pressure management are closely connected. Exposure to cold weather can lead to increased intracranial pressure due to vasoconstriction (the narrowing of blood vessels) and the body's natural response to cold stress. Proper winter gear plays a critical role in maintaining stable body temperature and preventing sudden fluctuations that could exacerbate symptoms.

However, those who have a shunt must be cautious about how winter hats and scarves fit around the head and neck. A shunt system, typically consisting of a catheter and valve, helps drain excess cerebrospinal fluid from the brain to another part of the body (such as the abdomen). Any external pressure on the shunt valve or tubing could potentially interfere with its function, leading to discomfort, increased pressure, or shunt malfunction. Additionally, tight or restrictive winter gear can worsen headaches, dizziness, or skin irritation for individuals with sensitive scalps or neurological conditions.

Challenges of Wearing Winter Gear with a Shunt

Before exploring solutions, it's important to understand the specific challenges that individuals with hydrocephalus or shunts may face when wearing winter hats and scarves:

1. **Pressure on the Shunt Site**: Shunts are typically placed in the head, with tubing that runs behind the ear or down the neck. Hats or scarves that are too tight can place direct pressure on the shunt valve, potentially disrupting its function or causing discomfort.
2. **Sensitive Scalp**: Many individuals with hydrocephalus experience scalp sensitivity, especially around the shunt site. This sensitivity can make wearing hats, especially tight-fitting ones, uncomfortable or even painful.

3. **Overheating and Sweating**: While warmth is important, overheating due to heavy or tightly woven hats can be problematic. Overheating can lead to sweating, which in turn can increase discomfort, trigger headaches, or contribute to skin irritation around the shunt site.

4. **Weight and Material of Winter Gear**: Heavier hats and scarves, especially those made of thick wool or bulky fabrics, can exert unnecessary pressure on the head and neck. These materials may also trap heat excessively, leading to discomfort or overheating.

5. **Mobility Issues**: Individuals with hydrocephalus may have difficulties with fine motor skills or coordination, which can make putting on and adjusting winter gear more challenging. Hats or scarves that are easy to put on, adjust, or remove are essential for managing comfort throughout the day.

Tips for Choosing Comfortable Winter Hats

Choosing the right hat is crucial for keeping warm without causing pressure on the head or shunt. Here are some key considerations when selecting a winter hat:

1. Look for Soft, Stretchy Materials

The material of the hat is one of the most important factors in ensuring comfort. Choose hats made from soft, stretchy fabrics that can conform to the shape of your head without exerting pressure.

- **Recommended Materials**: Hats made from lightweight, breathable fabrics like fleece, cotton, or soft acrylic are ideal. These materials provide warmth without being too heavy or restrictive.
- **Avoid Heavy Wool**: While wool is a great insulator, some types of wool hats can be too heavy or tight, causing discomfort on the scalp or around the shunt area. If you prefer wool, look for hats made from lightweight, merino wool, which is softer and more breathable.

2. Opt for Loose-Fitting or Adjustable Hats

A loose-fitting or adjustable hat allows for better control over the fit and reduces the risk of putting pressure on the shunt or sensitive areas of the scalp. Avoid hats that are too tight, as they can create pressure points.

- **Beanies and Slouchy Hats**: Beanies and slouchy hats are excellent options for individuals with hydrocephalus, as they offer a snug but flexible fit. Look for beanies that have some stretch but are not overly tight.
- **Hats with Adjustable Straps**: Some winter hats, such as fleece caps or trapper hats, come with adjustable straps or closures, allowing you to customize the fit around your head. This feature is particularly useful for accommodating changes in head size or sensitivity.

3. Consider Lightweight, Layered Options

Instead of wearing a single thick hat, consider wearing layers to stay warm without adding pressure to your head. A thin, breathable hat or headband worn underneath a looser hat can provide warmth without the bulk.

- **Thin, Breathable Base Layers**: You can wear a thin, breathable hat or skullcap made of moisture-wicking fabric under a looser winter hat. This combination allows for warmth without overheating or excessive pressure.
- **Headbands**: For those who want to avoid pressure on the top of the head or shunt area altogether, headbands made from fleece or wool are a great alternative. They keep your ears and forehead warm while leaving the top of your head free from pressure.

4. Choose Hats with Minimal Seams

Seams on hats can cause irritation, especially if they align with the shunt or sensitive parts of the scalp. Look for hats with minimal or flat seams to reduce the likelihood of discomfort.

- **Seamless or Flat-Seamed Hats**: Many athletic-style winter hats or fleece beanies are designed with flat seams or are seamless, which can be more comfortable for individuals with hydrocephalus or shunts.
- **Avoid Bulky or Ribbed Seams**: Bulky seams, especially around the edges of the hat, can cause pressure and discomfort, particularly if they press directly on the shunt tubing or valve.

5. Consider Weather-Appropriate Hats

For extremely cold or windy conditions, hats with additional features like ear flaps or wind-resistant linings can provide extra warmth without requiring a tight fit.

- **Hats with Ear Flaps**: Trapper hats or fleece-lined caps with ear flaps provide warmth for the ears and neck without needing to fit tightly over the entire head.
- **Wind-Resistant Linings**: Some winter hats come with windproof or water-resistant linings, which offer protection against harsh weather conditions. These hats can keep you warm without needing to be overly thick or heavy.

Tips for Choosing Comfortable Scarves

Scarves are essential for protecting your neck and chest from the cold, but they can also place pressure on the shunt tubing, especially if the shunt runs down the neck. Here are some tips for selecting scarves that provide warmth without causing discomfort:

1. Opt for Lightweight, Breathable Fabrics

Just like hats, scarves made from lightweight, breathable fabrics are less likely to cause discomfort or irritation around the shunt area.

- **Recommended Fabrics**: Choose scarves made from soft, lightweight materials such as fleece, cashmere, or cotton blends. These fabrics offer warmth without being too bulky or heavy.
- **Avoid Heavy Wool**: Thick, heavy wool scarves can place too much pressure on the neck and may cause overheating. If you prefer wool, opt for lightweight versions or wool blends that are softer and more breathable.

2. Avoid Tight, Wrapping Scarves

Scarves that are wrapped too tightly around the neck can place pressure on the shunt tubing and cause discomfort. Instead, look for looser-fitting scarves that can be draped comfortably.

- **Infinity Scarves**: Infinity scarves are a great option because they can be looped loosely around the neck without needing to be tied tightly. This reduces pressure on the neck while still providing warmth.
- **Shawl-Style Scarves**: Shawl-style scarves or wraps can be draped around the shoulders and chest without wrapping tightly around the neck. This is a good option for those who are particularly sensitive to pressure on the neck area.

3. Use Neck Gaiters for a Snug but Gentle Fit

Neck gaiters, also known as buffs or snoods, are versatile alternatives to traditional scarves. They provide warmth for the neck and can be pulled up to cover the lower face, but they do not need to be wrapped or tied.

- **Soft, Stretchy Gaiters**: Look for neck gaiters made from soft, stretchy materials like fleece or merino wool. These fabrics will provide warmth while allowing for a snug but gentle fit around the neck.
- **Adjustable Gaiters**: Some neck gaiters come with adjustable cords or toggles, allowing you to customize the fit. This can be particularly useful for ensuring that the gaiter does not place pressure on the shunt tubing.

4. Keep Scarves Loose Around the Neck

If you prefer traditional scarves, make sure to keep them loose and avoid tying them too tightly around the neck. A loosely draped scarf will still provide warmth without compressing the neck or shunt area.

- **Use a Single Loop**: Instead of wrapping the scarf multiple times around your neck, use a single loop and let the ends hang loosely. This will provide warmth without adding pressure to the neck.
- **Tuck Scarves Underneath Coats**: Tucking the ends of your scarf inside your coat can help keep it in place without the need to tie it tightly. This method also provides extra insulation by trapping warm air inside your coat.

Practical Tips for Comfort and Safety

In addition to choosing the right winter gear, there are practical steps you can take to ensure that your hats and scarves are worn comfortably without causing pressure or discomfort:

- **Check Fit Regularly**: Throughout the day, check the fit of your hat and scarf to ensure they are not placing too much pressure on your head or neck. Adjust them as needed to maintain comfort.
- **Rotate Winter Gear**: If you have multiple hats and scarves, rotate them regularly to prevent irritation in the same areas of your head or neck. This can help reduce the risk of developing pressure points or skin irritation.
- **Consult with Your Healthcare Provider**: If you experience discomfort or concerns about pressure on your shunt, consult with your healthcare provider for personalized advice on managing your winter gear. They may have specific recommendations based on the location and type of shunt you have.

Conclusion

Wearing winter gear comfortably is essential for individuals with hydrocephalus, particularly those with a shunt. The right hats and scarves can help you stay warm during the colder months while minimizing pressure on sensitive areas of the scalp and neck. By choosing soft, breathable fabrics, opting for loose-fitting or adjustable options, and being mindful of how your winter gear fits, you can enjoy the winter season without compromising comfort or shunt function.

With careful selection and attention to fit, wearing winter hats and scarves can be both practical and comfortable, allowing you to manage your cranial pressure while staying cozy during the winter months.

Chapter 6: Staying Hydrated in Cold Weather
The Importance of Hydration and Its Effect on Managing Hydrocephalus

Hydration is essential for everyone, but for individuals with hydrocephalus, maintaining proper fluid balance is particularly important. Hydrocephalus is characterized by an abnormal accumulation of cerebrospinal fluid (CSF) in the brain, and while hydration does not directly control CSF production or drainage, staying well-hydrated plays a crucial role in overall brain health and body function. Proper hydration can help regulate blood pressure, prevent headaches, reduce the risk of complications, and support the effective functioning of medical devices like shunts.

While hydration may seem less of a concern during cold weather than in the heat of summer, the winter season poses unique challenges to staying properly hydrated. Cold weather often suppresses the sensation of thirst, and people tend to drink less water during colder months, potentially leading to dehydration. Indoor heating systems can also dry out the air, increasing fluid loss through the skin and respiratory system. In this chapter, we will explore why hydration is important for individuals with hydrocephalus, how cold weather affects hydration, and practical strategies for staying hydrated during the winter months.

The Role of Hydration in Managing Hydrocephalus

Hydration impacts multiple systems in the body, and for individuals with hydrocephalus, maintaining an optimal fluid balance is important for several reasons:

1. Maintaining Intracranial Pressure (ICP)

Proper hydration helps regulate blood pressure and overall fluid balance in the body. Dehydration can cause the body to retain fluids, leading to an increase in blood pressure, which can subsequently affect intracranial pressure. Elevated ICP can exacerbate symptoms of hydrocephalus, such as headaches, nausea, dizziness, and visual disturbances.

Conversely, overhydration—while less common—can also contribute to fluid imbalances in the body. Therefore, it's essential to maintain a balanced level of hydration, where fluid intake is aligned with the body's needs.

2. Preventing Headaches

One of the most common symptoms associated with hydrocephalus is headaches, which can be triggered or worsened by dehydration. When the body becomes dehydrated, the brain loses water, leading to the shrinkage of brain tissue and increased pressure on the surrounding blood vessels. This can result in headaches that are more intense or prolonged, especially for those with hydrocephalus.

Staying hydrated helps prevent dehydration-induced headaches and may reduce the overall frequency and severity of headaches related to ICP fluctuations.

3. Supporting Shunt Function

Many individuals with hydrocephalus rely on a shunt system to help drain excess cerebrospinal fluid from the brain to another part of the body, typically the abdomen. While hydration doesn't directly impact the function of the shunt, it plays a critical role in maintaining overall fluid balance and preventing complications such as infection, which can affect the shunt.

Proper hydration helps keep bodily systems—including the immune system—functioning optimally, reducing the risk of infections that could compromise the shunt's effectiveness.

4. Maintaining Cognitive Function

Dehydration affects cognitive performance, which can be particularly concerning for individuals with hydrocephalus who may already experience cognitive difficulties. Even mild dehydration can impair attention, memory, and concentration. For those managing hydrocephalus, maintaining hydration is crucial for supporting mental clarity and reducing cognitive fatigue.

5. Regulating Body Temperature

Hydration is essential for regulating body temperature, particularly during physical activity or exposure to cold environments. In the winter, people may underestimate the importance of hydration when engaging in outdoor activities, such as walking or shoveling snow. However, even in cold weather, the body loses fluid through sweat and respiration, which can lead to dehydration if not replenished.

How Cold Weather Affects Hydration

Cold weather introduces several unique challenges when it comes to maintaining proper hydration:

1. Suppressed Thirst Response

In cold weather, the body naturally suppresses the sensation of thirst as part of its thermoregulation process. When exposed to cold temperatures, the body prioritizes conserving heat by constricting blood vessels, which reduces blood flow to the skin. This reduces the body's perceived need for water, even though fluid loss continues to occur through normal bodily functions like breathing, sweating, and urination.

As a result, people often feel less thirsty in cold weather and may not drink as much water as they need, leading to dehydration.

2. Increased Fluid Loss Through Respiration

When breathing in cold air, the body loses water as moisture is expelled through the breath. This process happens at a faster rate in cold weather than in warmer temperatures, as the air tends to be drier. The cold, dry air also causes the mucous membranes in the respiratory system to lose moisture more quickly, further contributing to fluid loss.

3. Dry Indoor Air

Indoor heating systems, which are commonly used during the winter months, create dry environments that can lead to dehydration. Heated indoor air causes the skin to lose moisture more rapidly, contributing to dehydration, even when individuals are not engaging in physical activity. The dry air can also lead to dry mouth, irritated sinuses, and cracked skin, all of which are signs of dehydration.

4. Sweating During Physical Activity

Even in cold weather, physical activity can lead to sweating. Outdoor activities such as walking, shoveling snow, or winter sports cause the body to lose fluids through sweat, especially if individuals are dressed in layers of clothing. However, because cold temperatures reduce the sensation of sweating, people may not realize they are losing water and may neglect to hydrate adequately.

Signs of Dehydration to Watch For

Recognizing the signs of dehydration is critical for managing hydrocephalus, particularly in cold weather when people may be less aware of their hydration levels. Common signs of dehydration include:

- **Dry Mouth or Throat**: A lack of moisture in the mouth or throat is one of the earliest signs of dehydration.
- **Dark-Colored Urine**: Dark yellow or amber-colored urine indicates that the body is not receiving enough water. Ideally, urine should be light yellow or clear.
- **Fatigue or Dizziness**: Dehydration can lead to feelings of fatigue, dizziness, or lightheadedness, particularly after physical activity.
- **Headaches**: Dehydration can trigger or worsen headaches, especially in individuals with hydrocephalus who are prone to ICP-related headaches.
- **Dry Skin**: Dry, flaky skin, or cracked lips are common signs of dehydration, especially in dry, cold environments.
- **Cognitive Difficulties**: Difficulty concentrating, forgetfulness, or confusion may also be linked to dehydration, as the brain needs adequate water to function optimally.

Practical Strategies for Staying Hydrated in Cold Weather

Staying hydrated during the winter months requires conscious effort, particularly since the body's natural thirst signals are diminished in the cold. Here are some practical strategies to ensure adequate hydration throughout the winter season:

1. Drink Water Regularly, Even When Not Thirsty

Because cold weather suppresses the sensation of thirst, it's important to drink water regularly, even if you don't feel thirsty. Set a goal to drink a certain amount of water each day, and make it a habit to sip water throughout the day rather than waiting until you feel thirsty.

- **Use a Water Bottle**: Carry a refillable water bottle with you throughout the day as a visual reminder to drink. Aim to drink small amounts of water consistently rather than trying to drink a large amount at once.
- **Set Hydration Goals**: Set specific hydration goals, such as drinking a glass of water every hour or ensuring you consume a certain number of ounces of water each day. This can help you stay on track with your hydration needs.

2. Incorporate Hydrating Foods

In addition to drinking water, consuming water-rich foods can help you stay hydrated. Many fruits and vegetables have high water content and can contribute to your overall fluid intake.

- **Water-Rich Foods**: Foods such as cucumbers, oranges, strawberries, watermelon, celery, and leafy greens are excellent sources of hydration. Incorporating these foods into your diet can provide additional fluids and nutrients.
- **Soups and Broths**: During the winter months, warm soups and broths are a great way to stay hydrated while also providing warmth and comfort. Clear broths, vegetable soups, and herbal teas can help replenish fluids while keeping you warm in cold weather.

3. Monitor Your Urine Color

One of the easiest ways to check your hydration status is by monitoring the color of your urine. As mentioned earlier, dark-colored urine is a sign of dehydration, while light yellow or clear urine indicates proper hydration.

- **Check Regularly**: Make it a habit to check the color of your urine, especially after waking up in the morning or after engaging in physical activity. If your urine is dark, it's a sign that you need to drink more water.

4. Use a Humidifier Indoors

Indoor heating systems can create dry air that contributes to dehydration. Using a humidifier in your home can help maintain moisture in the air and reduce the risk of dehydration caused by dry indoor environments.

- **Place Humidifiers in Key Areas**: Use a humidifier in areas where you spend the most time, such as the bedroom or living room. This can help prevent dry skin, dry mouth, and respiratory discomfort caused by dry air.

5. Drink Warm Beverages

During the winter, it's common to gravitate toward warm beverages to stay cozy. While some warm drinks, such as caffeinated coffee or tea, can contribute to dehydration, there are plenty of hydrating warm beverages that can help keep you hydrated.

- **Herbal Teas**: Herbal teas, such as chamomile, peppermint, or ginger tea, are hydrating and caffeine-free, making them a great option for staying hydrated in cold weather.
- **Warm Water with Lemon**: Drinking warm water with a slice of lemon is a simple and hydrating way to stay warm while replenishing fluids. The lemon adds a refreshing taste, and warm water is easier to drink when it's cold outside.

6. Limit Dehydrating Beverages

Certain beverages, such as alcohol and caffeinated drinks, can lead to dehydration. While it's fine to enjoy these beverages in moderation, it's important to be mindful of their diuretic effects, especially in cold weather when fluid loss may go unnoticed.

- **Moderate Caffeine Intake**: Caffeine acts as a diuretic, meaning it can increase urine output and contribute to dehydration. If you drink coffee or caffeinated tea, balance your intake with water or herbal teas to stay hydrated.
- **Limit Alcohol Consumption**: Alcohol also has a dehydrating effect, particularly if consumed in large quantities. If you plan to drink alcohol during holiday celebrations or social events, be sure to drink water alongside it to maintain hydration.

7. Stay Hydrated During Physical Activity

Even in cold weather, physical activity can cause fluid loss through sweat, so it's important to stay hydrated during and after exercise or outdoor activities.

- **Drink Water Before and After Activity**: Make it a habit to drink water before engaging in any physical activity, such as walking, shoveling snow, or winter sports. After the activity, replenish fluids by drinking water or a hydrating beverage.

Conclusion

Staying hydrated is crucial for individuals with hydrocephalus, as proper hydration helps regulate intracranial pressure, prevent headaches, support shunt function, and maintain cognitive function. While cold weather can suppress thirst and lead to unintentional dehydration, there are several practical strategies for ensuring adequate hydration during the winter months.

By drinking water regularly, incorporating water-rich foods into your diet, using a humidifier to combat dry indoor air, and monitoring your urine color, you can maintain proper hydration and reduce the risk of dehydration-related complications. Staying mindful of hydration throughout the winter will help support your overall health and well-being, allowing you to manage your hydrocephalus symptoms effectively while enjoying the colder months.

Chapter 7: Adapting to Travel Plans with Hydrocephalus
Handling Long-Distance Travel, Especially by Plane, Train, or Car

For individuals with hydrocephalus, long-distance travel presents a unique set of challenges. Hydrocephalus, a condition characterized by the abnormal accumulation of cerebrospinal fluid (CSF) in the brain, can lead to fluctuations in intracranial pressure (ICP). Changes in altitude, prolonged periods of sitting, disruptions in routine, and other factors associated with travel can exacerbate symptoms such as headaches, nausea, and dizziness, making it crucial to plan carefully. Whether traveling by plane, train, or car, individuals with hydrocephalus can benefit from strategies that help manage these challenges and ensure a safe, comfortable journey.

In this chapter, we will explore the potential effects of different modes of travel on individuals with hydrocephalus, outline the specific risks and considerations for each, and provide detailed tips on how to manage long-distance travel to minimize the impact on your condition.

The Impact of Travel on Hydrocephalus

Traveling, especially over long distances, can introduce physical and environmental stressors that may affect an individual with hydrocephalus. Here are some common factors that can influence symptoms during travel:

1. Altitude Changes

For those flying or traveling to higher elevations, changes in altitude can affect intracranial pressure. Higher altitudes mean lower atmospheric pressure, which can cause ICP to fluctuate. This can lead to symptoms like headaches, nausea, dizziness, or increased pressure in the head.

2. Prolonged Sitting and Immobility

Long periods of sitting, whether in an airplane, car, or train, can lead to reduced blood circulation and muscle stiffness. This can exacerbate headaches, cause discomfort in the neck and shoulders, and even contribute to an increase in ICP.

3. Disruption of Routine

Travel often means changes to daily routines, including medication schedules, sleep patterns, hydration levels, and meal times. For individuals managing hydrocephalus, maintaining a consistent routine is critical for managing symptoms. Disruptions can increase stress and trigger symptoms like fatigue or cognitive difficulties.

4. Dehydration

Travel, especially by air, can contribute to dehydration due to dry cabin air, changes in routine, and insufficient water intake. Dehydration can lead to increased ICP, headaches, and overall discomfort for those with hydrocephalus.

5. Stress and Fatigue

Travel can be stressful, whether due to long lines at airports, navigating unfamiliar places, or adhering to tight schedules. Emotional and physical stress, combined with travel fatigue, can worsen hydrocephalus symptoms. Managing stress is crucial for keeping symptoms under control.

Preparing for Travel with Hydrocephalus

The key to successful travel with hydrocephalus is preparation. Before embarking on your journey, take the time to prepare both physically and logistically to minimize the risk of symptom flare-ups. Here are important steps to take before traveling:

1. Consult with Your Healthcare Provider

Before making travel plans, consult with your neurologist or neurosurgeon. They can provide specific recommendations tailored to your condition and travel plans. Discuss the following:

- **Altitude Sensitivity**: If you're flying or traveling to a high-altitude location, ask whether you are at increased risk for complications related to altitude changes. Your healthcare provider may offer advice on managing altitude-related symptoms or suggest medications to control ICP.
- **Medications**: Ensure you have enough medication for the entire trip, including any extras in case of delays. Ask if any medications need to be adjusted based on your travel schedule, and request written documentation of your prescriptions, especially for international travel.
- **Shunt Functionality**: If you have a shunt to manage hydrocephalus, ensure that it is functioning properly before travel. Your healthcare provider may advise a check-up or imaging study (such as a CT scan or MRI) to verify that everything is in order before a long trip.

2. Pack an Emergency Travel Kit

Having a well-prepared travel kit can make the journey smoother and more comfortable. Your kit should include:

- **Medications**: Carry all essential medications in your carry-on luggage for easy access. Keep them in their original containers with prescription labels, especially when flying, to avoid issues with security.
- **Medical Documentation**: Carry a medical alert card or letter from your doctor explaining your condition and detailing any emergency protocols. This is particularly important if you are traveling internationally.
- **Pain Relief**: Pack over-the-counter pain relief, such as ibuprofen or acetaminophen, to manage headaches or other discomforts during travel.
- **Water Bottle**: A refillable water bottle is essential for staying hydrated during your trip, especially on flights where dehydration can occur more rapidly.
- **Snacks**: Bring healthy snacks, especially if you need to take medications with food or anticipate delays in meal service.
- **Comfort Items**: Consider packing a neck pillow, eye mask, and noise-canceling headphones to make the journey more comfortable and help manage sensory overload.

3. Plan for Rest and Recovery

Travel can be physically and mentally exhausting, especially for those managing hydrocephalus. Plan for rest periods throughout your journey and allow extra time for recovery once you arrive at your destination. Make sure your itinerary includes plenty of downtime to prevent overexertion.

Managing Air Travel with Hydrocephalus

Air travel is the most common form of long-distance travel, but it presents several unique challenges for individuals with hydrocephalus. Changes in cabin pressure, dehydration, and the long duration of flights can all contribute to symptom flare-ups. Here's how to manage air travel effectively:

1. Altitude and Cabin Pressure

The changes in cabin pressure during a flight can affect individuals with hydrocephalus, particularly if they are sensitive to changes in altitude. While modern airplanes are pressurized, the cabin pressure still equates to being at an altitude of about 6,000 to 8,000 feet, which can cause mild fluctuations in intracranial pressure.

Tips for Managing Cabin Pressure:

- **Stay Hydrated**: Drink plenty of water before and during the flight to combat the dehydrating effects of cabin air and help stabilize ICP. Avoid alcohol and caffeine, which can increase dehydration.
- **Use Pressure-Equalizing Earplugs**: Consider using earplugs designed to regulate pressure in your ears during takeoff and landing. These can help reduce discomfort related to altitude changes.
- **Move Around**: If you are on a long flight, make sure to get up and move around the cabin every hour or so. Walking and stretching can improve circulation and reduce the risk of blood clots, which are a concern during prolonged immobility.

2. Shunt Considerations During Air Travel

While air travel is generally safe for individuals with shunts, it's essential to remain vigilant about how your body feels during and after the flight.

Shunt-Related Precautions:

- **Monitor for Symptoms**: During the flight, be aware of symptoms such as severe headaches, nausea, vomiting, or visual disturbances, which could indicate changes in ICP. If you experience any of these symptoms, notify the flight crew immediately.
- **Carry Shunt Information**: If you have a programmable shunt, carry the programming card with you, as changes in pressure could potentially affect the shunt settings. In rare cases, a programmable shunt may need to be adjusted after a flight.

3. Tips for Long Flights

Long flights can be tiring and may disrupt your usual routine. Here are some additional tips to stay comfortable on long-haul flights:

- **Pre-Select Your Seat**: If possible, choose a seat that offers more legroom or easier access to the aisle, allowing you to stretch your legs and move around. A window seat may offer more privacy and allow you to rest undisturbed, while an aisle seat provides easy access for bathroom breaks.
- **Use a Neck Pillow**: A comfortable neck pillow can help support your neck and head, reducing strain during long flights.
- **Bring Comfort Items**: Pack an eye mask, blanket, or travel pillow to create a more relaxing environment and reduce sensory overload.

Managing Car Travel with Hydrocephalus

Car travel offers more flexibility than air travel, but long drives still come with their own challenges for individuals with hydrocephalus, such as limited movement, posture-related discomfort, and sensory overload from motion or traffic.

1. Take Frequent Breaks

Long periods of sitting can lead to discomfort, muscle stiffness, and increased ICP, so it's important to take regular breaks during road trips.

Break Suggestions:

- **Stretch and Move**: Every 1-2 hours, stop for a break to stretch, walk around, and change positions. Gentle stretching exercises can relieve tension and improve circulation.
- **Plan Rest Stops**: If you're driving long distances, plan your route with rest stops along the way. This allows you to rest, hydrate, and take any necessary medication.

2. Stay Comfortable in the Car

Maintaining comfort during long car rides can help prevent headaches, back pain, and other discomforts.

Comfort Tips:

- **Use Cushions and Pillows**: Bring a lumbar support cushion or seat pillow to reduce strain on your lower back and maintain good posture.
- **Adjust the Seat**: Make sure your car seat is adjusted for optimal comfort and support. Recline the seat slightly if it helps reduce pressure on your neck and shoulders.
- **Wear Comfortable Clothing**: Dress in loose, comfortable clothing that allows for easy movement and won't add pressure to sensitive areas like your head or neck.

3. Manage Motion Sickness

Some individuals with hydrocephalus may be more prone to motion sickness, which can trigger nausea, dizziness, and headaches during car travel.

Motion Sickness Management:

- **Focus on the Horizon**: If you're a passenger, try to sit in the front seat and focus on a fixed point on the horizon. This can help reduce motion sickness.
- **Use Anti-Nausea Remedies**: If you're prone to motion sickness, consider using over-the-counter anti-nausea medications or natural remedies like ginger tablets or acupressure wristbands.

Managing Train Travel with Hydrocephalus

Train travel can offer a more relaxed and spacious environment than air or car travel, but it still requires careful planning, especially for long journeys.

1. Move Around Frequently

Like air travel, train travel allows for easy movement throughout the cabin. Make sure to take advantage of this by walking around periodically to stretch your legs and improve circulation.

- **Walk Every Hour**: Take a short walk every hour to prevent stiffness and reduce the risk of blood clots.
- **Use Station Stops for Fresh Air**: If the train makes stops, step outside (when allowed) to get some fresh air and stretch.

2. Manage Comfort During the Ride

Train seats tend to be more spacious than airplane or car seats, but comfort is still essential for managing hydrocephalus symptoms during long journeys.

Comfort Suggestions:

- **Bring a Travel Pillow**: A travel pillow can support your neck during naps or rest periods. Consider bringing a blanket for added comfort.
- **Seat Selection**: If possible, reserve a window seat, which may provide more stability and reduce the risk of motion sickness.

Tips for International Travel

International travel requires additional planning, especially for individuals with hydrocephalus who may need access to medical care in unfamiliar locations.

1. Research Medical Facilities

Before traveling abroad, research the availability of medical facilities and neurology centers near your destination. This can help you prepare in case of an emergency.

- **Locate Nearest Hospitals**: Know the location of the nearest hospitals or emergency clinics, especially those with neurosurgical capabilities.
- **Travel Insurance**: Consider purchasing travel insurance that covers medical emergencies, including those related to hydrocephalus or shunt complications.

2. Prepare for Time Zone Changes

If traveling across time zones, adjusting your medication schedule may be necessary. Consult your healthcare provider about how to manage medication timing to prevent disruptions in your routine.

Conclusion

Traveling with hydrocephalus requires careful planning and attention to detail, but with the right strategies, you can enjoy your journey while minimizing the risk of symptom flare-ups. Whether traveling by plane, car, or train, it's essential to stay hydrated, maintain comfort, and plan for rest breaks to manage intracranial pressure and other hydrocephalus-related challenges.

By consulting with your healthcare provider, packing an emergency kit, staying mindful of altitude changes, and making comfort a priority, you can adapt to long-distance travel with confidence. Following these tips will help ensure a safe and enjoyable trip, allowing you to focus on the experience without compromising your health and well-being.

Chapter 8: Air Travel and Intracranial Pressure
Specific Strategies for Managing Air Pressure Changes During Flights

Air travel is a convenient and sometimes necessary mode of transportation, but for individuals with hydrocephalus, it presents unique challenges. Changes in cabin pressure during flights, particularly during ascent and descent, can cause fluctuations in intracranial pressure (ICP), which may exacerbate symptoms such as headaches, nausea, dizziness, and visual disturbances. Understanding how air pressure changes affect ICP and knowing how to manage these fluctuations are key to ensuring a safe and comfortable flight for individuals with hydrocephalus.

This chapter will provide a comprehensive guide on how air travel affects intracranial pressure and offer specific strategies to mitigate the impact of these pressure changes on individuals with hydrocephalus. By adopting these strategies, travelers can reduce discomfort and minimize the risk of symptom flare-ups during and after their flight.

Understanding Air Pressure and Its Effect on Hydrocephalus

Air pressure decreases as altitude increases, and when you fly, the airplane's cabin is pressurized to simulate the air pressure at approximately 6,000 to 8,000 feet above sea level. While this cabin pressurization helps reduce the effects of altitude, it still results in a lower atmospheric pressure than what you experience on the ground. For individuals with hydrocephalus, these changes in air pressure can affect the dynamics of cerebrospinal fluid (CSF) within the brain, leading to fluctuations in intracranial pressure.

The brain and the ventricles where CSF accumulates are sensitive to changes in pressure. As the external pressure decreases at higher altitudes, the body may respond with symptoms such as headaches, dizziness, and pressure sensations in the head. For those with hydrocephalus, especially those with shunts, these pressure changes can have a more pronounced impact, potentially affecting the function of the shunt or triggering a rise in ICP.

Potential Symptoms During Air Travel

Individuals with hydrocephalus may experience various symptoms related to intracranial pressure changes during air travel, particularly during takeoff, ascent, descent, and landing. Common symptoms include:

- **Headaches**: Often described as pressure-like or throbbing headaches, these can occur due to fluctuations in ICP.
- **Nausea and Vomiting**: The sensation of increased pressure or changes in CSF dynamics can lead to nausea, sometimes accompanied by vomiting.
- **Dizziness or Vertigo**: Changes in pressure can affect balance and lead to dizziness or a sensation of spinning (vertigo).
- **Visual Disturbances**: Blurred vision, double vision, or difficulty focusing can occur as a result of ICP fluctuations.

- **Ear Pressure and Discomfort**: Pressure changes during ascent and descent can cause discomfort in the ears, which may be intensified in individuals with hydrocephalus.

Specific Strategies for Managing Air Pressure Changes During Flights

While air travel poses certain challenges for individuals with hydrocephalus, there are several strategies that can help manage the impact of pressure changes and reduce the likelihood of symptoms during a flight.

1. Pre-Flight Preparation

Proper preparation is essential to managing intracranial pressure during air travel. Before your flight, take the following steps:

- **Consult with Your Healthcare Provider**: Before traveling, especially if this is your first time flying with hydrocephalus or after a recent shunt surgery, consult with your neurologist or neurosurgeon. They may recommend specific precautions or medications to manage ICP during the flight. If you have a programmable shunt, your doctor may provide instructions on how to monitor shunt settings and functionality before and after the flight.
- **Pack an Emergency Travel Kit**: Prepare a travel kit that includes any medications you may need, pain relievers for managing headaches, and medical documentation explaining your condition. This documentation should include details about your shunt (if applicable), current medications, and emergency contact information for your healthcare provider.
- **Stay Hydrated Before the Flight**: Dehydration can exacerbate the effects of altitude changes on intracranial pressure. Make sure to drink plenty of water in the days leading up to your flight to ensure that your body is well-hydrated before takeoff.

2. Managing Cabin Pressure During the Flight

Once on board, there are several strategies to help mitigate the effects of cabin pressure changes on intracranial pressure:

- **Use Pressure-Equalizing Earplugs**: Ear pressure during takeoff and landing can cause discomfort, particularly for individuals with hydrocephalus. Pressure-equalizing earplugs are designed to slow down the rate at which pressure changes in your ears, reducing discomfort during altitude changes. These earplugs can be worn during the entire flight but are especially helpful during takeoff and descent when pressure changes are most pronounced.
- **Hydrate During the Flight**: Cabin air is extremely dry, which can lead to dehydration and worsen symptoms related to ICP. Make sure to drink water regularly throughout the flight. Avoid alcohol and caffeinated beverages, as they can contribute to dehydration.
- **Move and Stretch Regularly**: Long periods of sitting can contribute to muscle stiffness and poor circulation, which may exacerbate headaches and pressure sensations. Try to move around the cabin and stretch every 1-2 hours during the flight. Walking to the restroom or doing simple in-seat stretches can help improve circulation and reduce the risk of discomfort.

3. Managing Symptoms During Takeoff and Landing

Takeoff and landing are the times when changes in cabin pressure are most rapid, making these phases of the flight particularly challenging for individuals with hydrocephalus. Here's how to manage symptoms during these critical times:

- **Practice Slow Breathing Techniques**: During takeoff and landing, practice deep, slow breathing to help relax your body and manage any anxiety or discomfort. Controlled breathing can help reduce the sensation of pressure in the head and prevent hyperventilation, which can worsen symptoms.
- **Chew Gum or Suck on Hard Candy**: Chewing gum or sucking on hard candy can help alleviate ear pressure by encouraging swallowing, which helps equalize pressure in the ears. This can reduce the discomfort associated with pressure changes and prevent the sensation of "plugged" ears during descent.
- **Use a Cold Compress for Headaches**: If you feel a headache coming on during takeoff or landing, consider using a cold compress or cold pack to help reduce the sensation of pressure in your head. You can ask the flight attendants for ice, which can be wrapped in a cloth and applied to the back of your neck or forehead to alleviate discomfort.

4. Post-Flight Recovery

Once the flight is over, it's important to give your body time to recover from the effects of air travel. Here are some post-flight strategies to help you feel better after landing:

- **Rehydrate**: After the flight, continue to drink plenty of water to replenish any fluids lost during the journey. Rehydrating will help reduce headaches, fatigue, and the effects of any dehydration that may have occurred during the flight.
- **Rest and Relax**: Air travel can be physically and mentally exhausting, especially for individuals with hydrocephalus. Plan for some downtime after your flight to rest and recover. If possible, schedule your travel so that you have time to relax at your destination before engaging in any strenuous activities.
- **Monitor Symptoms**: Keep an eye on how you feel after the flight. If you experience persistent or worsening symptoms, such as severe headaches, vomiting, or confusion, contact your healthcare provider immediately. These could be signs of elevated ICP or shunt malfunction and may require medical attention.

Special Considerations for Individuals with Shunts

For individuals with hydrocephalus who have a shunt in place to regulate cerebrospinal fluid, there are additional considerations to keep in mind during air travel:

1. Programmable Shunts

Programmable shunts allow for adjustments to the flow of CSF based on the patient's needs. While air travel is generally safe for individuals with programmable shunts, cabin pressure changes can, in rare cases, affect the shunt's settings.

- **Carry a Shunt Programming Card**: If you have a programmable shunt, carry your programming card with you during travel. This card provides important information about your shunt's settings and can be useful if you need medical assistance while traveling.
- **Monitor Shunt Function**: After the flight, be aware of any signs that your shunt may not be functioning properly, such as a persistent headache, changes in vision, or nausea. If you suspect that your shunt settings have been affected by the flight, contact your healthcare provider, who can check the shunt and adjust its settings if necessary.

2. Shunt Malfunction Symptoms

In rare cases, air pressure changes may contribute to shunt malfunction. It's important to be aware of the signs of shunt malfunction, which can include:

- Severe headaches that do not improve with rest or medication
- Nausea and vomiting
- Unexplained drowsiness or difficulty waking up
- Blurred or double vision
- Difficulty walking or coordinating movements
- Personality changes or irritability

If you experience any of these symptoms during or after your flight, seek immediate medical attention.

Tips for International Air Travel

International air travel involves longer flight times and additional complexities, such as crossing time zones and dealing with potential language barriers when seeking medical care. Here are some additional tips for managing international travel with hydrocephalus:

- **Plan for Jet Lag**: Crossing time zones can disrupt your sleep patterns, which may affect how you manage hydrocephalus symptoms. Prepare for jet lag by adjusting your sleep schedule before departure and staying hydrated throughout your trip.
- **Research Medical Facilities at Your Destination**: Before you travel internationally, research the medical facilities at your destination. Identify hospitals or clinics that have neurology or neurosurgery departments in case you need medical assistance during your trip.
- **Carry a Letter from Your Doctor**: When traveling internationally, it's important to carry a letter from your healthcare provider that explains your condition, any medications you are taking, and the specifics of your shunt (if applicable). This letter can help local medical professionals understand your needs in case of an emergency.

Conclusion

Air travel can present unique challenges for individuals with hydrocephalus, but with proper preparation and symptom management, it is possible to fly safely and comfortably. Understanding how air pressure changes affect intracranial pressure, consulting with your healthcare provider, and implementing strategies such as staying hydrated, using pressure-equalizing earplugs, and taking breaks to stretch during the flight can help mitigate the effects of cabin pressure changes.

Whether you're flying domestically or internationally, these strategies will help ensure that your air travel experience is as smooth and symptom-free as possible. By preparing ahead of time and paying close attention to your body's signals during the flight, you can minimize the risk of symptom flare-ups and enjoy your journey with confidence.

Chapter 9: Managing Travel Fatigue
Reducing Exhaustion During Holiday Trips and How to Pace Yourself

Travel, particularly during the busy holiday season, can be physically and mentally exhausting for anyone, but for individuals with hydrocephalus, managing travel fatigue is especially important. Hydrocephalus, a condition characterized by an accumulation of cerebrospinal fluid (CSF) in the brain, often leads to symptoms such as headaches, cognitive difficulties, and fatigue. The additional strain of long journeys, whether by car, train, or airplane, can exacerbate these symptoms, making travel more challenging. Learning how to pace yourself and manage travel fatigue effectively can significantly reduce the physical and emotional toll of holiday trips, ensuring a more comfortable and enjoyable experience.

In this chapter, we will explore the causes of travel fatigue, its effects on individuals with hydrocephalus, and provide practical strategies for reducing exhaustion and pacing yourself during holiday trips. By following these tips, you can manage your energy levels, minimize symptom flare-ups, and make the most of your travel experience.

Understanding Travel Fatigue and Its Impact on Hydrocephalus

Travel fatigue is a combination of physical and mental exhaustion that results from long periods of sitting, changes in routine, disrupted sleep, and the stress associated with navigating unfamiliar environments. For individuals with hydrocephalus, travel fatigue can be particularly debilitating, as it can worsen existing symptoms, such as headaches, cognitive fatigue, and sensitivity to sensory stimuli like noise and light.

Here are some common factors that contribute to travel fatigue:

- **Prolonged Sitting**: Long hours of sitting during car, train, or air travel can lead to muscle stiffness, reduced blood circulation, and discomfort, all of which can contribute to fatigue.
- **Disrupted Routine**: Travel often involves changes to your normal routine, such as irregular sleep patterns, altered meal times, and disruptions to medication schedules. These changes can cause physical and mental fatigue, especially for those who rely on a consistent routine to manage hydrocephalus symptoms.
- **Stress**: The stress of traveling—whether it's navigating airports, dealing with delays, or coordinating plans with others—can lead to emotional exhaustion. Stress is a known trigger for many symptoms of hydrocephalus, including headaches and cognitive difficulties.
- **Sensory Overload**: Crowded airports, busy train stations, and noisy public transportation can overwhelm the senses, leading to mental fatigue and increasing the risk of headaches or dizziness.
- **Sleep Disruption**: Travel often involves disruptions to your usual sleep schedule, whether due to time zone changes (jet lag), early departures, or difficulty sleeping in unfamiliar envi-

ronments. Poor sleep can amplify fatigue and make it harder to manage hydrocephalus symptoms.

The Effects of Travel Fatigue on Individuals with Hydrocephalus

For individuals with hydrocephalus, travel fatigue can manifest in several ways, including:

- **Increased Headaches**: Prolonged sitting, dehydration, stress, and disrupted sleep can all contribute to headaches, which are one of the most common symptoms of hydrocephalus. Travel fatigue can lead to an increase in the frequency or severity of headaches, especially if intracranial pressure fluctuates during travel.
- **Cognitive Fatigue**: Individuals with hydrocephalus often experience cognitive challenges, such as difficulty concentrating, memory lapses, or confusion. Travel fatigue can exacerbate these issues, making it harder to focus or think clearly during the trip.
- **Emotional Exhaustion**: Stress and fatigue can lead to feelings of irritability, anxiety, or emotional burnout. For individuals with hydrocephalus, this emotional strain can be particularly challenging, as emotional well-being is closely tied to managing physical symptoms.
- **Physical Weakness**: Fatigue can also manifest as physical weakness, making it more difficult to engage in activities such as walking, lifting luggage, or standing for long periods.

Practical Strategies for Reducing Travel Fatigue

To minimize travel fatigue and manage hydrocephalus symptoms effectively, it's essential to pace yourself and adopt strategies that support your physical and mental well-being during the journey. Here are some detailed, practical tips to help reduce exhaustion during holiday trips.

1. Plan Your Itinerary with Rest in Mind

The key to managing travel fatigue is to pace yourself by building rest and recovery time into your travel itinerary. Avoid overloading your schedule with back-to-back activities or long travel days that don't allow for breaks.

- **Schedule Rest Periods**: Whether you're traveling by car, train, or airplane, plan for regular rest breaks throughout the journey. On road trips, schedule stops every 1-2 hours to stretch, walk, and rehydrate. If you're flying, try to take short walks during the flight or stretch in your seat to prevent muscle stiffness.
- **Avoid Overbooking Your Day**: When planning holiday activities, avoid cramming too much into one day. Allow yourself time to rest between activities, and consider prioritizing key events while leaving room for downtime.
- **Plan Recovery Time Upon Arrival**: After a long trip, schedule time to rest and recover before engaging in any major activities. If you arrive at your destination in the afternoon or evening, plan for a low-key evening to recuperate.

2. Maintain Your Routine as Much as Possible

Maintaining a consistent routine during travel can help reduce the impact of fatigue and keep hydrocephalus symptoms in check. Here's how to adapt your routine while traveling:

- **Stick to Your Medication Schedule**: Ensure that you take your medications at the same time each day, even when traveling across time zones. Use a medication reminder app or set alarms to help you stay on track.
- **Follow Your Usual Sleep Patterns**: Try to maintain a consistent sleep schedule, even if you're in a different time zone. If possible, adjust your sleep patterns gradually in the days leading up to your trip to minimize the impact of jet lag.
- **Eat Regular Meals**: Irregular meal times can lead to drops in energy levels and contribute to fatigue. Pack healthy snacks for the journey, and plan your meals in advance to ensure that you're eating at regular intervals.

3. Manage Stress to Prevent Fatigue

Traveling during the holidays can be stressful, but managing stress effectively can reduce fatigue and prevent symptom flare-ups. Here are some strategies for minimizing stress while traveling:

- **Arrive Early**: Whether you're catching a flight or departing for a road trip, give yourself plenty of time to avoid the stress of rushing. Arriving early at the airport or train station can help reduce anxiety and give you time to relax before your journey begins.
- **Use Relaxation Techniques**: Practice relaxation techniques, such as deep breathing exercises, mindfulness, or meditation, to help calm your mind during stressful moments. These techniques can be particularly helpful during crowded or chaotic travel situations, such as airport security checks or delays.
- **Delegate Tasks**: If you're traveling with others, don't hesitate to delegate tasks such as handling luggage, coordinating travel arrangements, or navigating busy environments. Let others take the lead when necessary to conserve your energy.

4. Stay Hydrated to Combat Fatigue

Dehydration can worsen travel fatigue and exacerbate hydrocephalus symptoms, such as headaches and cognitive difficulties. Staying well-hydrated is essential, especially when flying, as cabin air can be extremely dry.

- **Drink Water Regularly**: Carry a refillable water bottle and sip water throughout the journey. If you're flying, be mindful of the dry cabin air and aim to drink at least 8 ounces of water for every hour of flight time. Avoid excessive caffeine or alcohol, as both can contribute to dehydration.

- **Hydrate Before Bed**: If your trip disrupts your sleep schedule, staying hydrated before bed can help reduce the risk of waking up with a headache or feeling sluggish. Keep a glass of water next to your bed to stay hydrated throughout the night.

5. Prioritize Comfortable Clothing and Travel Accessories

Wearing comfortable, loose-fitting clothing and using ergonomic travel accessories can reduce physical discomfort and help prevent fatigue during long trips.

- **Wear Layers**: Dress in layers to accommodate changes in temperature throughout your journey. Being too hot or too cold can contribute to fatigue, so choose clothing that allows you to easily adjust your comfort level.
- **Use Travel Pillows and Cushions**: Bring a neck pillow, lumbar support cushion, or travel blanket to stay comfortable during long periods of sitting. Proper support can prevent muscle tension and reduce fatigue.
- **Wear Comfortable Shoes**: If your trip involves walking through airports, train stations, or tourist destinations, wear comfortable, supportive shoes that reduce strain on your feet and legs.

6. Move and Stretch Regularly

Prolonged sitting can lead to muscle stiffness and reduced circulation, both of which contribute to travel fatigue. Regular movement and stretching can help alleviate these issues and keep you feeling more energized.

- **Stretch In Your Seat**: Even if you're unable to walk around during your journey, you can perform simple stretches in your seat. Try ankle rolls, shoulder shrugs, and gentle neck stretches to reduce tension and improve circulation.
- **Walk Whenever Possible**: If you're on a long flight or train ride, take advantage of opportunities to walk around the cabin. If you're on a road trip, schedule regular stops to get out of the car and stretch your legs.

7. Get Quality Sleep During Travel

Sleep is one of the most critical factors in managing travel fatigue. While it can be challenging to get quality sleep on a plane, train, or in a hotel, there are strategies you can use to improve your chances of restful sleep:

- **Use Sleep Aids**: Bring an eye mask, earplugs, or noise-canceling headphones to block out light and noise during the trip. These sleep aids can create a more restful environment, whether you're on a flight or in a hotel room.
- **Consider Melatonin for Jet Lag**: If you're traveling across time zones, consider using melatonin supplements to help regulate your sleep-wake cycle. Consult with your healthcare provider before taking melatonin or any other sleep aid.

• **Create a Relaxing Pre-Sleep Routine**: Establish a calming bedtime routine, even while traveling. This could include reading, listening to calming music, or practicing deep breathing exercises. Avoid screens and electronic devices before bed, as blue light can interfere with sleep.

Conclusion

Managing travel fatigue is essential for individuals with hydrocephalus, particularly during the busy holiday season when travel can be both physically and mentally exhausting. By pacing yourself, maintaining a consistent routine, staying hydrated, and prioritizing rest, you can reduce the impact of fatigue and prevent the worsening of hydrocephalus symptoms during your journey.

With careful planning and attention to your physical and emotional needs, you can enjoy your holiday trips while minimizing exhaustion and discomfort. These strategies will help you manage your energy levels effectively, ensuring that your travels are as stress-free and enjoyable as possible.

Chapter 10: Packing Medical Essentials

A Checklist of Medical Supplies, Shunt Records, and Emergency Contacts for Holiday Travel

Traveling during the holiday season can be exciting, but for individuals with hydrocephalus, it requires careful planning, especially when it comes to packing essential medical supplies. Whether you are traveling by car, train, or plane, having the right medical supplies on hand can ensure a safe and comfortable journey, prevent complications, and provide peace of mind. Proper preparation is particularly important for those who rely on a shunt system to manage cerebrospinal fluid (CSF), as travel introduces the possibility of emergency situations, such as shunt malfunction, dehydration, or changes in intracranial pressure (ICP). Packing a well-thought-out medical kit can help you handle any challenges that arise during your trip.

In this chapter, we will provide an extensive checklist of medical supplies, shunt records, emergency contacts, and other essential items that should be packed for holiday travel. By following this guide, you can ensure that you are prepared for any situation that may arise during your trip, allowing you to travel with confidence and focus on enjoying the holiday season.

Why Packing Medical Essentials is Crucial for Individuals with Hydrocephalus

Travel introduces various stressors that can affect individuals with hydrocephalus, including changes in routine, dehydration, altitude fluctuations, and long periods of sitting. These factors can impact intracranial pressure and lead to symptom flare-ups such as headaches, nausea, dizziness, and fatigue. For those with a shunt, there is also a risk of shunt malfunction or infection, both of which may require immediate medical attention.

Having the right medical supplies and documentation can help you:

1. **Manage Symptoms**: Essential medications, pain relievers, and hydration aids can help you manage symptoms like headaches, nausea, and dizziness that may arise during travel.
2. **Respond to Emergencies**: In the event of a medical emergency, such as shunt malfunction, having medical documentation and emergency contacts readily available can expedite your access to appropriate care.
3. **Maintain Routine**: Packing medications, assistive devices, and comfort items can help you stick to your usual routine while traveling, reducing the risk of complications or symptom exacerbation.
4. **Ensure Comfort**: Items such as neck pillows, compression socks, and comfortable clothing can alleviate physical discomfort during long trips, helping to reduce travel fatigue.

Packing Medical Essentials: A Detailed Checklist

1. Medications

Ensuring that you have enough medication to last throughout your trip is critical for managing hydrocephalus symptoms and maintaining your routine. Follow these tips when packing your medications:

- **Pack a Sufficient Supply**: Bring enough medication to last for the entire trip, plus an additional supply in case of travel delays. If you are traveling internationally or over long distances, it's wise to pack at least a week's worth of extra medication.
- **Keep Medications in Original Packaging**: Always carry your medications in their original packaging, with the prescription label clearly visible. This is particularly important for air travel, as it helps avoid issues during security screening.
- **Organize Medication with a Pill Case**: Use a daily pill organizer to keep track of your medication schedule during travel. This is especially helpful for longer trips or if you need to take medications at specific times each day.
- **Carry Medications in Your Carry-On Bag**: If you are flying, keep all medications in your carry-on bag to ensure they are easily accessible and avoid the risk of losing them with checked luggage.
- **Bring a Prescription List**: Carry a list of all your current medications, including dosages and instructions. This can be useful if you need to replace a lost or damaged prescription while traveling.

2. Pain Relief and Symptom Management

Hydrocephalus symptoms such as headaches, nausea, and dizziness can flare up during travel due to changes in routine, altitude, or cabin pressure (on planes). Be sure to pack over-the-counter remedies to help manage these symptoms:

- **Pain Relievers**: Pack pain relievers such as ibuprofen, acetaminophen, or aspirin to manage headaches or other aches and pains. Be mindful of dosage recommendations and any interactions with other medications you are taking.
- **Anti-Nausea Medications**: If you are prone to nausea, pack over-the-counter or prescription anti-nausea medications (such as dimenhydrinate, meclizine, or ondansetron) to help alleviate symptoms during travel.
- **Motion Sickness Aids**: If you are traveling by car, plane, or boat and experience motion sickness, consider packing remedies such as motion sickness wristbands, ginger tablets, or acupressure bands.
- **Cold or Hot Compresses**: Pack a small, portable cold or hot compress to help relieve headaches or neck stiffness. Some compresses can be activated without the need for refrigeration or heating, making them ideal for travel.

3. Hydration and Nutrition

Staying hydrated is crucial for managing hydrocephalus symptoms, particularly during air travel or when traveling to high-altitude destinations. Here's what to pack to ensure proper hydration and nutrition during your trip:

- **Reusable Water Bottle**: Bring a refillable water bottle that you can use throughout your journey. If you are flying, empty the bottle before going through security and refill it after passing through screening.
- **Electrolyte Tablets or Powders**: Electrolyte supplements can help replenish lost fluids and prevent dehydration. Pack electrolyte tablets or powder packets to mix with water during your trip, especially if you will be engaging in physical activity or traveling in hot climates.
- **Healthy Snacks**: Bring non-perishable, healthy snacks such as granola bars, trail mix, or dried fruit. This ensures you have access to nutritious food during long travel days or if meal options are limited.

4. Shunt Records and Medical Documentation

If you have a shunt, it's important to carry detailed records of your shunt system, as well as medical documentation explaining your condition. In case of an emergency, this information can be invaluable to healthcare providers who may not be familiar with your medical history.

- **Shunt Information Card**: Carry a card or document that provides key details about your shunt, including the type of shunt, the manufacturer, the model, and the settings (if you have a programmable shunt). This card should also include information about your shunt's placement and any previous surgeries.
- **Medical Alert ID**: Wear a medical alert bracelet or necklace that indicates you have hydrocephalus and a shunt. This can be helpful in emergencies when you may be unable to communicate your medical condition.
- **Doctor's Letter**: Bring a letter from your healthcare provider explaining your condition, your treatment plan, and any specific instructions in case of an emergency. This is especially important for international travel, where healthcare providers may be unfamiliar with your medical background.
- **Medical History Summary**: Carry a summary of your medical history, including any past surgeries, hospitalizations, and treatments related to hydrocephalus. Include contact information for your primary care physician and neurosurgeon.

5. Emergency Contacts

Having quick access to emergency contacts is essential when traveling, particularly if you experience symptoms of shunt malfunction or other medical issues. Make sure you have the following information readily available:

- **Primary Healthcare Provider**: Include the name, phone number, and email address of your primary care physician or neurologist. Ensure that this contact information is stored in your phone and written on a physical card in your medical kit.
- **Neurosurgeon Contact Information**: If you have a shunt, carry the contact information for your neurosurgeon, as well as the hospital or clinic where your surgeries were performed. This is particularly important for international travel, where local doctors may need to consult with your neurosurgeon in case of an emergency.
- **Family and Caregiver Contacts**: Include contact information for close family members or caregivers who are familiar with your medical history and can assist in an emergency. Make sure this information is stored in both your phone and a physical document.
- **Local Emergency Services**: Research the emergency contact numbers for the country or region you are visiting, especially if you are traveling internationally. In some countries, the emergency number is not 911, so it's important to know the correct number in advance.

6. Travel Insurance and Medical Coverage

Travel insurance that includes medical coverage can provide peace of mind, especially if you are traveling abroad. Be sure to review your travel insurance policy and pack the necessary documentation:

- **Travel Insurance Policy**: Pack a copy of your travel insurance policy, including the policy number, coverage details, and contact information for the insurance provider. Ensure that your policy covers medical emergencies, including hospitalization, emergency surgery, and medical evacuation if needed.
- **Proof of Health Insurance**: Bring your health insurance card and any relevant documentation that proves your coverage, both for domestic and international travel. If your health insurance provider offers international coverage, familiarize yourself with the steps required to access care while abroad.

7. Assistive Devices and Comfort Items

Long journeys can be physically taxing, especially for individuals with hydrocephalus who may experience fatigue, headaches, or discomfort during travel. Be sure to pack assistive devices and comfort items to make the trip more manageable:

- **Neck Pillow and Lumbar Support**: A supportive neck pillow or lumbar cushion can reduce neck and back strain during long periods of sitting. Choose a travel-friendly option that is lightweight and easy to pack.
- **Compression Socks**: Compression socks can improve circulation and reduce the risk of swelling during long flights or car trips. This is particularly important for preventing blood clots, which can be a concern during extended periods of immobility.
- **Eye Mask and Earplugs**: An eye mask and noise-canceling earplugs or headphones can help block out light and noise, making it easier to rest during travel. These items are especially useful during flights or train rides.
- **Blanket or Shawl**: A lightweight blanket or shawl can provide warmth and comfort during long trips. Some travel blankets are designed to fold compactly for easy packing.

Packing Tips for Air Travel

If you are flying, there are additional considerations for packing your medical essentials. Follow these tips to ensure a smooth and stress-free experience at the airport:

- **TSA Screening**: Familiarize yourself with the Transportation Security Administration (TSA) rules regarding medications and medical devices. You are allowed to bring medications in your carry-on, even if they are liquid or exceed the usual size limits for liquids. Be prepared to inform the TSA agent about your medical condition and any shunt-related devices.
- **Keep Medical Supplies Easily Accessible**: Pack your medical supplies in a carry-on bag that you can easily access during the flight. This ensures that essential items such as medications, pain relief, and medical documentation are within reach at all times.
- **Label Your Medical Bag**: Clearly label your medical bag with your name, contact information, and a description of its contents. This can be helpful in case the bag is misplaced or if you need to explain its contents to airport staff.

Conclusion

For individuals with hydrocephalus, packing the right medical essentials is a critical part of preparing for holiday travel. By assembling a well-organized kit that includes medications, shunt records, medical documentation, emergency contacts, and comfort items, you can ensure that you are fully prepared to manage your condition while on the go. Whether you are traveling domestically or internationally, taking the time to pack thoughtfully will help reduce stress, prevent complications, and allow you to enjoy the holiday season with greater peace of mind.

By following this detailed checklist and tailoring it to your specific medical needs, you can focus on the joy of the journey and the celebration, knowing that you are prepared for whatever challenges may arise during your travels.

Chapter 11: Handling Delayed Travel with Hydrocephalus
Managing Stress and Cranial Pressure During Unexpected Travel Delays

Travel delays are an unavoidable part of holiday travel, whether you're facing flight cancellations, train delays, or traffic jams. For anyone, these disruptions can be frustrating and stressful, but for individuals with hydrocephalus, managing delays requires extra attention and planning. Travel delays can disrupt carefully managed routines, cause physical discomfort, and increase stress levels—all of which can exacerbate hydrocephalus symptoms such as headaches, fatigue, nausea, and fluctuations in intracranial pressure (ICP).

In this chapter, we will explore how travel delays affect individuals with hydrocephalus and provide detailed strategies for managing both the physical and emotional challenges that may arise. By staying prepared, focusing on stress management, and prioritizing self-care during these unexpected situations, you can reduce the impact of delays on your health and well-being.

How Travel Delays Affect Individuals with Hydrocephalus

Travel delays can disrupt your plans in several ways, and for individuals with hydrocephalus, the consequences of these delays can be more severe due to their condition. Understanding how delays can affect your body and brain can help you prepare and manage these situations more effectively.

1. Disruption of Routine

One of the primary challenges of managing hydrocephalus is maintaining a consistent routine, including regular medication schedules, meals, hydration, and rest. Unexpected delays—whether they occur at the airport, on the road, or while waiting for a train—can throw off this routine. Disruptions to your medication schedule can lead to missed doses, while irregular meals and dehydration can worsen symptoms such as headaches or cognitive difficulties.

2. Increased Stress

Travel delays are inherently stressful, and for individuals with hydrocephalus, stress is a significant trigger for symptom flare-ups. Emotional stress activates the body's fight-or-flight response, increasing heart rate, blood pressure, and overall tension. This can lead to elevated intracranial pressure (ICP), which may cause headaches, nausea, and dizziness. Managing stress is essential for maintaining stable ICP and reducing the risk of symptom exacerbation.

3. Extended Periods of Sitting and Inactivity

Long periods of sitting, especially in uncomfortable environments such as crowded airport lounges or train stations, can contribute to muscle stiffness, poor circulation, and increased ICP. For individuals with hydrocephalus, sitting still for extended periods can lead to physical discomfort, back pain, and worsening headaches.

4. Sensory Overload

Airports, train stations, and other public spaces can be noisy, bright, and crowded—conditions that can overwhelm the senses. For individuals with hydrocephalus, sensory overload can trigger headaches, cognitive fatigue, or emotional stress, especially during prolonged delays.

5. Dehydration and Hunger

Delays can interfere with your ability to access food and water regularly, especially in situations where restaurants, shops, or food services are limited. Dehydration and hunger can quickly lead to a drop in energy levels, increase feelings of discomfort, and exacerbate hydrocephalus-related symptoms such as headaches and fatigue.

Practical Strategies for Managing Stress and Cranial Pressure During Delays

While travel delays are unpredictable, there are several strategies that can help you manage the stress and physical discomfort that arise when your plans are unexpectedly disrupted. By preparing in advance and focusing on self-care, you can reduce the impact of delays on your condition.

1. Stay Calm and Focus on What You Can Control

The first and most important step in managing travel delays is to stay calm and focus on what you can control. Stress is a significant trigger for hydrocephalus symptoms, so managing your emotional response to delays is essential.

- **Practice Deep Breathing**: When faced with a delay, practice slow, deep breathing to calm your nervous system and reduce the physical effects of stress. Inhale deeply through your nose for four counts, hold for four counts, and exhale slowly through your mouth for four counts. This can help lower your heart rate and blood pressure, reducing the risk of elevated ICP.
- **Focus on the Present Moment**: Mindfulness techniques, such as focusing on the present moment and avoiding catastrophizing, can help reduce anxiety during travel delays. Instead of worrying about how long the delay will last, focus on taking care of your immediate needs, such as staying hydrated and comfortable.
- **Take Breaks from the Situation**: If possible, step away from crowded or noisy environments, such as airport lounges or waiting areas. Find a quieter spot to sit, rest, and gather your thoughts. This can help reduce sensory overload and give you a mental break from the stress of the delay.

2. Maintain Your Medication Schedule

Keeping up with your medication schedule during travel delays is crucial for managing hydrocephalus symptoms. Here's how to stay on track:

- **Set Reminders**: Use your phone or a medication reminder app to set alarms for when it's time to take your medication. This will help ensure that you don't miss doses, even if you're distracted by the delay.
- **Carry Medications in Your Carry-On Bag**: Always keep your medications in your carry-on luggage or personal bag, rather than in checked luggage. This ensures that you have immediate access to your medications, even if your checked bags are delayed or lost.
- **Prepare for Extended Delays**: When traveling, always pack extra medication in case of unexpected delays. For example, if your trip is delayed by a full day or more, having an additional day's worth of medication can prevent gaps in your treatment.

3. Stay Hydrated and Nourished

Dehydration and hunger are common issues during travel delays, especially when access to food and water is limited. Both can contribute to headaches, fatigue, and worsened hydrocephalus symptoms, so it's essential to prioritize hydration and nourishment:

- **Carry a Refillable Water Bottle**: Bring a refillable water bottle with you and fill it regularly throughout your trip. Many airports and train stations have water fountains or bottle-filling stations, making it easy to stay hydrated. Aim to drink small amounts of water regularly to maintain hydration, especially if you are flying.
- **Pack Healthy Snacks**: Bring non-perishable, healthy snacks such as granola bars, nuts, dried fruit, or whole-grain crackers. These snacks can help maintain your energy levels and prevent drops in blood sugar if food options are limited during a delay.
- **Avoid Dehydrating Beverages**: During delays, it can be tempting to consume caffeinated or alcoholic beverages, but both can contribute to dehydration. Instead, stick to water or hydrating drinks like herbal teas or electrolyte-enhanced water.

4. Move and Stretch Regularly

Sitting for long periods in cramped or uncomfortable conditions can lead to muscle stiffness, poor circulation, and increased ICP. Make it a priority to move and stretch regularly during delays:

- **Walk Around**: If you're stuck in an airport or train station, take periodic walks around the terminal or waiting area. Even short walks can improve circulation, reduce muscle tension, and help alleviate discomfort.
- **Stretch in Your Seat**: If walking isn't possible, perform simple stretches while seated. Stretch your neck, shoulders, and legs to relieve tension. Gentle ankle rolls and shoulder shrugs can improve blood flow and reduce stiffness.
- **Use a Neck Pillow or Cushion**: If you anticipate sitting for a long time, bring a neck pillow or lumbar cushion to support your back and neck. This can help prevent strain and discomfort, especially during prolonged periods of inactivity.

5. Manage Sensory Overload

Busy travel hubs can be overwhelming, especially when you're dealing with delays. The noise, crowds, and bright lights can contribute to sensory overload and worsen symptoms such as headaches or cognitive fatigue. Here's how to manage sensory overload during travel delays:

- **Use Noise-Canceling Headphones**: Noise-canceling headphones can help block out the background noise of airports or train stations, providing a more peaceful environment. You can also use them to listen to calming music, audiobooks, or guided meditations to help reduce stress.

- **Wear Sunglasses**: If you're sensitive to bright lights, consider wearing sunglasses indoors. This can reduce eye strain and help prevent headaches caused by harsh lighting in public spaces.
- **Take Sensory Breaks**: When you feel overwhelmed by noise or crowds, find a quiet place where you can rest and recover. Many airports have designated quiet areas or lounges that provide a more relaxing environment. If none are available, consider stepping outside for some fresh air, weather permitting.

6. Practice Self-Care and Relaxation Techniques

Self-care is especially important during travel delays, as stress and discomfort can take a toll on your physical and emotional well-being. Incorporating relaxation techniques into your routine can help you stay calm and manage symptoms:

- **Meditation or Mindfulness**: Practicing mindfulness or meditation can help you stay centered during stressful situations. Focus on your breathing, practice gratitude, or use guided meditation apps to help calm your mind and reduce anxiety.
- **Progressive Muscle Relaxation**: Progressive muscle relaxation involves tensing and then slowly relaxing each muscle group in your body, starting from your toes and working your way up to your head. This technique can reduce physical tension and promote relaxation, helping to alleviate discomfort during delays.
- **Reading or Listening to Music**: Bring a book, e-reader, or music player to help distract yourself from the stress of delays. Engaging in a relaxing activity can improve your mood and take your mind off the inconvenience.

7. Plan for Sleep During Extended Delays

If your delay stretches into hours—or even overnight—finding a way to rest and sleep is essential for managing fatigue and preventing headaches or cognitive issues. Sleep deprivation can exacerbate hydrocephalus symptoms, so it's important to prioritize rest during long delays:

- **Bring a Travel Pillow and Blanket**: Pack a neck pillow, blanket, or shawl to help make resting more comfortable, even in airport chairs or train station benches.
- **Use an Eye Mask and Earplugs**: To block out light and noise, use an eye mask and earplugs, especially if you're trying to sleep in a busy environment. Noise-canceling headphones or earplugs can create a more peaceful setting for rest.
- **Find a Quiet Spot**: Look for quiet areas or designated rest zones in the airport or station where you can relax. Some airports have sleeping pods, lounges, or areas with more comfortable seating.

Recognizing Signs of Elevated Intracranial Pressure During Delays

For individuals with hydrocephalus, travel delays can sometimes lead to symptoms of elevated ICP due to stress, dehydration, or inactivity. It's important to be aware of these symptoms so that you can take action if they occur:

- **Persistent or Worsening Headaches**: A headache that becomes more intense or doesn't respond to pain relief could be a sign of elevated ICP.
- **Nausea and Vomiting**: Feeling nauseous or experiencing vomiting without a clear cause may indicate a rise in intracranial pressure.
- **Visual Disturbances**: Blurred vision, double vision, or difficulty focusing can be symptoms of increased pressure in the brain.
- **Dizziness or Balance Issues**: If you feel dizzy or unsteady on your feet, it could be related to changes in ICP.
- **Cognitive Difficulties**: Confusion, memory problems, or trouble concentrating may signal that your ICP is rising.

If you experience any of these symptoms during a travel delay, it's important to rest, hydrate, and try to alleviate stress. If symptoms persist or worsen, seek medical attention immediately.

Preparing for Future Delays

While no one can predict when or how long travel delays will last, being prepared for the possibility can help you manage them more effectively. Here are a few steps you can take to prepare for future delays:

- **Keep an Emergency Kit Ready**: Pack an emergency kit that includes medications, snacks, water, a neck pillow, noise-canceling headphones, and any other essentials that will help you stay comfortable during a delay.
- **Research Airports and Stations in Advance**: Before your trip, familiarize yourself with the layout of the airports, train stations, or bus terminals you'll be passing through. Knowing where to find rest areas, food options, and quieter spots can help you manage delays more effectively.
- **Have a Plan for Extended Delays**: Consider what you'll do if you face an extended delay, such as booking a hotel room for the night or contacting family or friends for support. Having a plan in place can reduce anxiety and help you navigate longer disruptions with confidence.

Conclusion

Travel delays are an inevitable part of holiday travel, but for individuals with hydrocephalus, they can present unique challenges. Managing stress, maintaining hydration, and sticking to your medication schedule are essential for preventing symptom flare-ups and ensuring a comfortable journey, even when unexpected disruptions occur.

By staying prepared with medical essentials, practicing relaxation techniques, and focusing on self-care, you can handle delays with greater ease and reduce the impact on your health and well-being. Ultimately, being proactive and adaptable during travel delays will help ensure that your holiday trip is as smooth and enjoyable as possible, despite any unexpected detours along the way.

Chapter 12: Food and Diet Tips for Holiday Dinners

How to Maintain a Diet That Helps Regulate Intracranial Pressure During Holiday Feasts

Holiday dinners are often filled with rich, indulgent foods and drinks that can be hard to resist. However, for individuals with hydrocephalus, maintaining a healthy diet that supports the regulation of intracranial pressure (ICP) is critical. Certain foods and beverages can exacerbate hydrocephalus symptoms by causing dehydration, inflammation, or fluctuations in blood pressure—all of which can affect ICP. That said, with mindful choices, you can still enjoy holiday feasts while managing your health.

In this chapter, we will explore the relationship between diet and intracranial pressure, highlight which foods to choose or avoid during holiday gatherings, and provide practical tips for maintaining a balanced and supportive diet. By following these guidelines, you can indulge in holiday meals while minimizing the risk of symptom flare-ups and staying in control of your condition.

Understanding the Impact of Diet on Intracranial Pressure

For individuals with hydrocephalus, maintaining proper intracranial pressure is essential to preventing symptoms such as headaches, nausea, dizziness, and cognitive difficulties. Diet plays a key role in regulating ICP by influencing blood pressure, hydration levels, and inflammation in the body. Certain foods can exacerbate hydrocephalus symptoms by causing fluid retention, increasing blood pressure, or leading to dehydration, while other foods can help maintain stability and support overall brain health.

Here are some ways diet affects intracranial pressure:

1. **Salt and Fluid Retention**: Foods high in sodium can cause the body to retain fluids, leading to an increase in blood pressure, which in turn can raise ICP. This is particularly concerning for individuals with hydrocephalus, as high ICP can trigger headaches and other symptoms.

2. **Hydration Levels**: Dehydration is a major factor that can lead to fluctuations in ICP. Staying properly hydrated is crucial, especially during the holidays when festive foods and drinks may lead to fluid loss or imbalances.

3. **Caffeine and Alcohol**: Both caffeine and alcohol act as diuretics, meaning they can lead to dehydration by increasing urine output. Excessive consumption of these beverages can contribute to dehydration, which can worsen symptoms such as headaches and cognitive fatigue.

4. **Inflammation and Processed Foods**: Highly processed foods, particularly those containing unhealthy fats and sugars, can promote inflammation in the body, which can contribute to increased ICP and overall discomfort. A diet rich in anti-inflammatory foods can help support brain health and reduce the risk of flare-ups.

Key Nutritional Considerations for Managing Intracranial Pressure

Before diving into specific tips for holiday dinners, it's important to understand the key nutritional considerations for managing hydrocephalus and regulating ICP. The following factors should guide your food and beverage choices during holiday gatherings:

- **Hydration**: Staying hydrated is essential for maintaining stable ICP. Drink plenty of water throughout the day, especially if you're consuming foods that are high in sodium or alcohol.
- **Moderate Sodium Intake**: High sodium intake can lead to fluid retention and increased blood pressure, both of which can raise ICP. Choose low-sodium foods when possible and be mindful of portion sizes when consuming salty dishes.
- **Limit Alcohol and Caffeine**: Alcohol and caffeine can dehydrate the body and contribute to ICP fluctuations. Moderation is key—enjoy these beverages in small amounts, and make sure to drink water alongside them.
- **Choose Whole Foods**: A diet rich in whole, unprocessed foods—such as fruits, vegetables, whole grains, lean proteins, and healthy fats—can help support overall brain health and prevent inflammation.
- **Prioritize Anti-Inflammatory Foods**: Foods rich in antioxidants, omega-3 fatty acids, and other anti-inflammatory compounds can help reduce inflammation and support brain function. Incorporating these foods into your holiday meals can help mitigate some of the effects of more indulgent treats.

Foods to Limit or Avoid During Holiday Dinners

Holiday dinners often feature rich, flavorful dishes that are high in salt, sugar, and unhealthy fats. While it's fine to enjoy these foods in moderation, some should be limited or avoided to prevent a spike in ICP. Here's a list of foods and drinks to be cautious about during holiday gatherings:

1. High-Sodium Foods

- **Processed Meats**: Ham, bacon, sausage, and other cured or smoked meats are often staples at holiday dinners, but they tend to be high in sodium. Choose smaller portions or opt for lower-sodium alternatives when available.
- **Cheese and Cheese-Based Dishes**: Cheese, particularly aged varieties, can be high in sodium. Cheesy casseroles, dips, and platters are common during the holidays but can contribute to fluid retention and increased ICP.
- **Canned Soups and Sauces**: Many soups, gravies, and sauces served at holiday dinners are made with canned or pre-packaged ingredients, which often contain high levels of sodium. Consider homemade versions with reduced sodium, or use herbs and spices to enhance flavor without added salt.

2. Sugary Foods

- **Desserts and Sweets**: Pies, cakes, cookies, and other holiday desserts are often loaded with sugar, which can contribute to inflammation and spikes in blood sugar levels. While it's fine to indulge in a sweet treat, be mindful of portion sizes and balance sugary foods with healthier options.
- **Sugary Beverages**: Soft drinks, fruit punches, and cocktails made with sugary mixers can cause rapid spikes in blood sugar, leading to energy crashes and inflammation. Opt for water, herbal teas, or drinks made with low-sugar alternatives.

3. Fried or Greasy Foods

- **Fried Appetizers and Sides**: Fried foods, such as fried chicken, potatoes, or appetizers like mozzarella sticks, are common at holiday feasts but are high in unhealthy fats that can contribute to inflammation and poor circulation. Limit your intake of these foods to avoid discomfort and fatigue.
- **Creamy or Butter-Laden Dishes**: Many traditional holiday dishes, such as mashed potatoes, stuffing, or casseroles, are made with generous amounts of butter or cream, which are high in saturated fats. These dishes can be enjoyed in moderation but should not dominate your meal.

4. Alcohol and Caffeinated Beverages

- **Alcohol**: While a glass of wine or a holiday cocktail may be tempting, excessive alcohol consumption can lead to dehydration, which worsens ICP-related symptoms. If you choose to drink alcohol, be sure to alternate with water and limit yourself to one or two drinks.
- **Caffeinated Drinks**: Coffee, tea, and soft drinks contain caffeine, which can act as a diuretic and lead to fluid loss. If you drink caffeinated beverages during the holiday dinner, balance them with plenty of water.

Foods to Include in Your Holiday Meals

Fortunately, there are plenty of delicious, nutrient-rich foods you can enjoy during holiday dinners that support brain health, reduce inflammation, and help regulate ICP. Incorporating these foods into your holiday meals can help you maintain a balanced diet while still enjoying festive favorites:

1. Hydrating Foods

- **Fruits and Vegetables**: Many fruits and vegetables have high water content and are rich in essential vitamins and minerals. Serve a colorful salad or vegetable platter alongside heavier dishes to add hydration and nutrients to your meal. Hydrating options include cucumbers, bell peppers, celery, watermelon, and oranges.
- **Broth-Based Soups**: Opt for broth-based soups instead of creamy, heavy varieties. A vegetable or chicken broth soup can be a lighter starter that helps keep you hydrated.

2. Anti-Inflammatory Foods

- **Omega-3-Rich Foods**: Omega-3 fatty acids have powerful anti-inflammatory properties and support brain health. Foods such as salmon, walnuts, flaxseeds, and chia seeds are excellent sources of omega-3s. If available, incorporate a salmon dish or sprinkle walnuts and flaxseeds on salads and side dishes.
- **Berries**: Berries such as blueberries, strawberries, and raspberries are rich in antioxidants and anti-inflammatory compounds. Serve them as part of a fruit platter or as a topping for lighter desserts.
- **Leafy Greens**: Dark leafy greens such as spinach, kale, and Swiss chard are loaded with vitamins, minerals, and antioxidants that support overall health and reduce inflammation. Incorporate these greens into salads, side dishes, or soups.

3. Low-Sodium Options

- **Fresh Proteins**: Instead of processed meats, opt for fresh, lean proteins such as roasted turkey, grilled chicken, or baked fish. These are lower in sodium and provide essential nutrients such as protein and omega-3s.
- **Herbs and Spices**: Use herbs and spices to season your food instead of relying on salt. Fresh herbs such as parsley, rosemary, thyme, and garlic can add flavor without contributing to fluid retention. Spices such as turmeric and ginger also have anti-inflammatory properties.

4. Healthy Fats

- **Avocados**: Avocados are a great source of healthy monounsaturated fats, which support brain health and reduce inflammation. Add slices of avocado to salads or serve guacamole as a dip for vegetable platters.
- **Olive Oil**: Use olive oil as a substitute for butter or margarine in cooking and baking. Olive oil is rich in healthy fats and antioxidants, making it a better choice for regulating blood pressure and inflammation.

5. Whole Grains

- **Quinoa, Brown Rice, and Whole-Grain Breads**: Whole grains provide fiber, which supports digestion and helps prevent blood sugar spikes that can contribute to fatigue. Serve whole grains as a side dish or opt for whole-grain bread instead of white bread for holiday stuffing.

Practical Tips for Managing Your Diet During Holiday Dinners

Navigating holiday dinners can be challenging, especially when there are many tempting dishes and drinks on the table. Here are some practical tips to help you maintain a balanced diet while enjoying holiday meals:

1. Plan Ahead

Before attending a holiday dinner, think about your dietary needs and plan how you'll navigate the meal. Consider bringing a healthy dish to share, such as a vegetable platter, salad, or whole-grain side dish. This ensures that you have a nutritious option available if the menu is heavy on rich, salty, or fried foods.

2. Portion Control

Portion control is key to enjoying holiday favorites without overindulging. Instead of piling your plate high with every dish, take smaller portions of high-sodium or high-fat foods and balance them with healthier options like vegetables, whole grains, and lean proteins.

3. Stay Hydrated

Make hydration a priority during the holiday meal. Drink a glass of water before sitting down to eat, and continue to sip water throughout the dinner. This will help prevent dehydration and reduce the likelihood of headaches or increased ICP.

4. Listen to Your Body

Pay attention to how your body feels during the meal. If you start to feel full or experience discomfort, stop eating and take a break. It's important to avoid overeating, as large meals can cause a spike in blood pressure and contribute to ICP fluctuations.

5. Balance Indulgence with Moderation

Holiday meals are meant to be enjoyed, so it's perfectly fine to indulge in your favorite holiday dishes. However, balance indulgence with moderation by focusing on smaller portions and balancing heavier foods with lighter, nutrient-dense options. For example, if you indulge in a slice of pie, pair it with fresh fruit or a small salad to balance the meal.

Conclusion

Holiday dinners can be a time of indulgence and celebration, but for individuals with hydrocephalus, it's essential to maintain a diet that helps regulate intracranial pressure and supports overall brain health. By being mindful of your food and beverage choices, focusing on hydration, and incorporating nutrient-dense, anti-inflammatory foods into your meals, you can enjoy the holiday season while minimizing the risk of symptom flare-ups.

With careful planning and a balanced approach, you can savor the flavors of holiday feasts without compromising your well-being. By following these dietary guidelines, you can maintain control over your condition and continue to celebrate the holidays with joy and confidence.

Chapter 13: Alcohol and Hydrocephalus

Understanding the Effects of Alcohol on Those with Hydrocephalus and Safe Consumption Guidelines

The holiday season and other social events often involve the consumption of alcohol, but for individuals with hydrocephalus, drinking alcohol requires careful consideration. Alcohol can have significant effects on the brain and body, and for those managing hydrocephalus, it may exacerbate symptoms, interfere with medications, or increase the risk of complications such as dehydration and fluctuations in intracranial pressure (ICP). While it may be possible to enjoy alcohol in moderation, understanding its potential risks and effects is essential for making informed decisions.

In this chapter, we will explore how alcohol affects individuals with hydrocephalus, how it influences ICP, and the specific risks involved. We will also provide guidelines for safe alcohol consumption to help you navigate social situations while minimizing the risk of symptom flare-ups and health complications.

How Alcohol Affects the Brain and Body

Alcohol has a range of effects on the brain and body, and its impact can vary based on factors such as age, weight, overall health, and existing medical conditions. For individuals with hydrocephalus, the effects of alcohol can be more pronounced due to the brain's altered fluid dynamics and the use of treatments such as shunts.

Here are the primary ways alcohol interacts with the brain and body, which are relevant to those with hydrocephalus:

1. Dehydration and Intracranial Pressure

Alcohol is a diuretic, meaning it increases urine production and leads to fluid loss. For individuals with hydrocephalus, dehydration can cause a range of symptoms, including headaches, dizziness, and cognitive difficulties, and may affect ICP. Adequate hydration is essential for regulating ICP, and alcohol's dehydrating effects can disrupt this balance, leading to a rise in pressure inside the skull.

When the body is dehydrated, the brain tissue can shrink slightly, pulling away from the skull and causing discomfort. This process can lead to a condition known as "brain dehydration," which is particularly dangerous for individuals with hydrocephalus, as it can exacerbate existing pressure imbalances and trigger headaches or other symptoms.

2. Impact on Cognitive Function

Alcohol is a central nervous system depressant that affects brain function, slowing down communication between brain cells. For individuals with hydrocephalus, who may already experience cognitive challenges such as memory problems, difficulty concentrating, or slowed thinking, alcohol can further impair cognitive function. Even moderate amounts of alcohol can interfere with your ability to think clearly, make decisions, or react quickly—skills that are already compromised for some individuals with hydrocephalus.

3. Risk of Interference with Medications

Many individuals with hydrocephalus take medications to manage symptoms, prevent seizures, or regulate fluid balance. Alcohol can interfere with the effectiveness of these medications, either by reducing their efficacy or by amplifying side effects. Common medications used by people with hydrocephalus, such as anticonvulsants or diuretics, can interact with alcohol, leading to dizziness, drowsiness, or impaired coordination. Mixing alcohol with these medications may also increase the risk of dangerous side effects.

4. Increased Risk of Falls and Injuries

For those with hydrocephalus, maintaining balance and coordination can already be a challenge. Alcohol can impair motor skills and slow reflexes, increasing the risk of falls and injuries. Even a small amount of alcohol can significantly impair coordination, making it difficult to walk steadily, navigate stairs, or avoid obstacles. For individuals with shunts, falls or head injuries can be particularly dangerous, as they may lead to shunt malfunction or other complications.

5. Potential for Increased Intracranial Pressure

Alcohol affects blood flow and can lead to changes in blood pressure, which in turn can impact intracranial pressure. Drinking alcohol dilates blood vessels, which increases blood flow to the brain. In individuals with hydrocephalus, this increase in blood flow can contribute to raised ICP, triggering symptoms such as headaches, nausea, or visual disturbances. In some cases, excessive drinking can cause ICP to rise to dangerous levels, leading to more serious complications.

6. Delayed Effects and Hangovers

The aftereffects of alcohol consumption, particularly hangovers, can be especially challenging for individuals with hydrocephalus. Hangovers are typically characterized by dehydration, headaches, fatigue, nausea, and cognitive difficulties—symptoms that overlap with those of hydrocephalus. The combination of a hangover and hydrocephalus symptoms can make the day after drinking particularly unpleasant and difficult to manage.

Safe Alcohol Consumption Guidelines for Individuals with Hydrocephalus

While alcohol consumption is not entirely off-limits for individuals with hydrocephalus, it should be approached with caution. If you choose to drink, it's important to follow safe consumption guidelines to minimize the risk of adverse effects. Here are some key recommendations to help you enjoy alcohol safely and responsibly:

1. Consult with Your Healthcare Provider

Before consuming alcohol, it's essential to consult with your healthcare provider, especially if you have hydrocephalus. Your doctor can provide specific recommendations based on your medical history, the type of treatment you're receiving (such as shunt placement), and any medications you're taking. In some cases, your doctor may advise you to avoid alcohol entirely, particularly if you are taking medications that interact negatively with alcohol.

2. Limit Alcohol Intake

Moderation is key when it comes to alcohol consumption, particularly for individuals with hydrocephalus. Excessive drinking can increase the risk of dehydration, raise ICP, and impair cognitive function. Here are some general guidelines for limiting alcohol intake:

- **Stick to One Drink or Less**: For most individuals with hydrocephalus, limiting alcohol to one drink (or less) per occasion is advisable. One drink is generally considered to be:
  - 12 ounces of beer (5% alcohol)
  - 5 ounces of wine (12% alcohol)
  - 1.5 ounces of distilled spirits (40% alcohol)
- **Pace Yourself**: Sip your drink slowly and space it out over time to give your body a chance to process the alcohol. Drinking too quickly can overwhelm your system and increase the likelihood of symptoms such as dizziness, headaches, or nausea.
- **Alternate with Water**: To combat dehydration, alternate alcoholic drinks with water. For every alcoholic beverage you consume, drink a glass of water to help maintain hydration levels and minimize the risk of ICP fluctuations.

3. Stay Hydrated

As alcohol dehydrates the body, it's crucial to stay hydrated before, during, and after drinking. Proper hydration helps regulate ICP and reduces the risk of alcohol-related symptoms such as headaches, dizziness, or cognitive fatigue. Here's how to maintain hydration while drinking:

- **Hydrate Before Drinking**: Make sure you're well-hydrated before consuming alcohol. Drink water or an electrolyte beverage in the hours leading up to a social event to ensure your body is in good balance.

- **Drink Water Between Alcoholic Beverages**: As mentioned earlier, alternate each alcoholic drink with a glass of water. This can slow down your alcohol consumption and help prevent dehydration.
- **Hydrate After Drinking**: Before going to bed, drink plenty of water to help your body re-hydrate after consuming alcohol. This can reduce the severity of hangover symptoms the next day.

4. Eat Before and During Drinking

Drinking alcohol on an empty stomach can lead to faster absorption of alcohol into the bloodstream, increasing the likelihood of dizziness, impaired judgment, and other symptoms. Eating before and during alcohol consumption can help slow the absorption process and minimize its impact on your body.

- **Eat a Balanced Meal**: Before consuming alcohol, eat a meal that includes healthy fats, protein, and complex carbohydrates. This can help stabilize blood sugar levels and reduce the risk of feeling lightheaded or unwell after drinking.
- **Snack During Drinking**: Continue to eat light snacks while drinking to maintain your energy levels and slow alcohol absorption. Nuts, cheese, whole-grain crackers, and vegetables with hummus are good snack options.

5. Avoid Mixing Alcohol with Medications

If you take medications to manage hydrocephalus or related symptoms, it's important to avoid mixing them with alcohol unless your healthcare provider has given you specific guidance. Many medications, including anticonvulsants, sedatives, and certain pain relievers, can interact negatively with alcohol, leading to heightened side effects such as drowsiness, confusion, or impaired coordination.

- **Check Labels and Consult Your Doctor**: Always read the labels of your medications to check for alcohol-related warnings. If you're unsure about whether it's safe to drink alcohol while on a particular medication, consult your doctor or pharmacist.

6. Know Your Limits and Recognize Symptoms

It's important to know your body's limits when it comes to alcohol consumption. If you notice any of the following symptoms after drinking, it may be a sign that your body is reacting negatively to the alcohol, and you should stop drinking immediately:

- **Severe Headache**: A sudden or intense headache could indicate a spike in ICP. If this occurs after drinking, stop consuming alcohol and hydrate immediately. Seek medical attention if the headache persists or worsens.

- **Dizziness or Confusion**: If you feel lightheaded, dizzy, or disoriented after consuming alcohol, it's best to stop drinking and rest. These symptoms may be a sign that your body is dehydrated or that your ICP is fluctuating.
- **Nausea or Vomiting**: If you experience nausea or vomiting after drinking, it could be a sign that alcohol is affecting your digestive system or increasing your ICP. In this case, stop drinking, hydrate, and rest.

7. Have a Plan for Safe Transportation

If you plan to drink alcohol during a social event, always have a plan for getting home safely. Alcohol can impair your judgment, coordination, and reaction time, making it unsafe to drive or operate machinery. Arrange for a designated driver, use a ride-sharing service, or take public transportation to ensure you get home without risking injury to yourself or others.

Conclusion

For individuals with hydrocephalus, alcohol consumption comes with unique risks that must be carefully managed. Alcohol's dehydrating effects, its impact on cognitive function, and its potential to raise intracranial pressure make it important to approach drinking with caution. By following safe consumption guidelines—such as limiting alcohol intake, staying hydrated, eating before drinking, and avoiding medication interactions—you can reduce the risk of alcohol-related complications and still enjoy social events responsibly.

Ultimately, the decision to consume alcohol is a personal one, and it's important to prioritize your health and well-being. By understanding how alcohol affects your body and taking steps to minimize its impact, you can make informed choices that allow you to participate in holiday celebrations and other social gatherings while maintaining control over your condition.

Chapter 14: Dealing with Overstimulation at Family Gatherings
Techniques to Avoid Sensory Overload During Loud or Busy Events

Family gatherings, especially during the holiday season, are filled with joy, laughter, and connection. However, they can also be overwhelming, particularly for individuals with hydrocephalus who may be more sensitive to overstimulation. The noise, bright lights, crowded spaces, and constant activity at family events can trigger sensory overload, leading to symptoms such as headaches, dizziness, fatigue, and emotional distress. Sensory overload can also exacerbate hydrocephalus-related symptoms, making it difficult to enjoy social gatherings.

In this chapter, we will explore how overstimulation affects individuals with hydrocephalus and provide detailed techniques to help you manage sensory overload during family gatherings. By implementing these strategies, you can navigate loud or busy events more comfortably while maintaining your well-being and enjoying time with loved ones.

Understanding Sensory Overload and Its Impact on Hydrocephalus

Sensory overload occurs when the brain becomes overwhelmed by excessive sensory input—such as noise, lights, movement, and social interactions. For individuals with hydrocephalus, the brain's ability to process and filter sensory information may already be compromised due to the condition's effects on the brain and its fluid dynamics. This makes people with hydrocephalus more vulnerable to sensory overload in environments that are loud, chaotic, or visually stimulating.

Here are some of the ways sensory overload can affect individuals with hydrocephalus:

1. Increased Intracranial Pressure (ICP)

Overstimulation, especially when combined with emotional stress, can raise ICP, leading to symptoms such as headaches, nausea, and dizziness. The increased sensory input requires the brain to work harder to process information, which can contribute to fluctuations in ICP.

2. Headaches and Cognitive Fatigue

Sensory overload can trigger or worsen headaches, which are a common symptom of hydrocephalus. The brain's effort to manage excessive noise, bright lights, or movement can lead to cognitive fatigue, making it difficult to concentrate, think clearly, or engage in conversations.

3. Emotional Stress and Irritability

The sensory demands of a busy family gathering can lead to emotional distress, including feelings of anxiety, frustration, or irritability. For individuals with hydrocephalus, these emotional responses can further exacerbate physical symptoms such as increased ICP or fatigue.

4. Difficulty Communicating and Socializing

When the brain is overwhelmed by sensory input, it can become challenging to focus on conversations, follow social cues, or respond appropriately in social situations. This can make socializing at family gatherings more difficult and contribute to feelings of isolation or frustration.

Techniques for Managing Sensory Overload at Family Gatherings

While family gatherings can be overstimulating, there are several techniques you can use to manage sensory overload and prevent symptom flare-ups. By planning ahead and practicing mindfulness during events, you can enjoy the social interaction without overwhelming your brain and body.

1. Plan for Breaks and Downtime

One of the most effective ways to prevent sensory overload is to schedule breaks and allow yourself downtime during family gatherings. Stepping away from the noise and activity gives your brain time to recover and reset, reducing the risk of overstimulation.

- **Designate Quiet Time**: Before attending the event, plan specific times when you'll step away to rest. This might be every hour or so, depending on how long the event lasts. Use these breaks to sit in a quiet room, take a short walk outside, or find a peaceful space to relax.
- **Communicate Your Needs**: Let your family know in advance that you may need to take occasional breaks during the gathering. This helps set expectations and reduces any pressure you might feel to stay engaged with the group at all times.

2. Use Sensory Management Tools

There are a variety of tools that can help you manage sensory input during busy or loud family events. These tools can reduce the impact of noise, light, and movement, helping to prevent sensory overload.

- **Noise-Canceling Headphones**: Noise-canceling headphones can be a lifesaver in loud environments. You can use them to block out background noise while listening to calming music, audiobooks, or white noise. This can help create a more peaceful environment for your brain, even when the room is bustling.
- **Earplugs**: If you don't want to wear headphones, consider using discreet earplugs to reduce noise levels. Earplugs are especially useful in environments with loud conversations, music, or clattering dishes, and they can help protect you from sensory overload without drawing attention.
- **Sunglasses or Tinted Glasses**: Bright lights, flashing decorations, or sunlight streaming through windows can contribute to visual overload. Wearing sunglasses or tinted glasses indoors can help reduce the intensity of lighting and prevent eye strain. If you're sensitive to certain lighting conditions, such as fluorescent lights, tinted glasses may also help.
- **Weighted Blanket or Vest**: For some individuals, deep pressure can have a calming effect on the nervous system. A weighted blanket or vest can help you feel grounded and provide relief from the constant sensory input around you. Consider using a weighted blanket during rest breaks or when sitting in a quieter part of the room.

3. Create a Sensory-Friendly Environment

If you have some control over the environment—such as if you're hosting or attending a gathering at a close relative's home—you can make adjustments to reduce sensory triggers and create a more sensory-friendly space.

- **Choose a Quiet Room**: If possible, identify a quieter room or area of the home where you can retreat if the main gathering space becomes too loud or chaotic. This room can serve as a refuge for breaks, providing a calm and peaceful space to rest.
- **Adjust Lighting**: Bright, harsh lighting can contribute to sensory overload. Dim the lights in the room or use soft lighting from lamps or string lights to create a more soothing atmosphere. Avoid flashing or strobe lights, which can be especially triggering for individuals with hydrocephalus or sensitivity to light.
- **Limit Background Noise**: If you're hosting the event or have influence over the setup, try to minimize background noise. For example, avoid playing loud music or having the TV on during the gathering, as these can add to the overall sensory input in the room.

4. Set Boundaries and Limit Social Interaction

Social interactions can be mentally taxing, especially when there are many conversations happening at once. Setting boundaries on how much socializing you engage in can help prevent cognitive fatigue and keep your energy levels up.

- **Engage in Smaller Groups**: Instead of trying to participate in large group conversations, opt for one-on-one or small group interactions. These conversations are easier to follow and less overwhelming. Additionally, speaking to fewer people at once allows you to focus on the conversation without distractions.
- **Limit Social Engagement**: It's okay to step back from socializing if you start to feel fatigued or overwhelmed. You don't have to be "on" the whole time. Let your family know if you need a break from conversations and allow yourself the time to recharge before re-engaging.
- **Take Short Walks or Get Fresh Air**: Stepping outside for a few minutes of fresh air can be a great way to reset and recover from sensory overload. A short walk outside or a moment of quiet can help you feel calmer and more refreshed.

5. Use Mindfulness and Breathing Techniques

Mindfulness and breathing exercises are powerful tools for calming the nervous system and reducing the effects of sensory overload. These techniques can help you stay grounded, centered, and in control when the environment becomes overwhelming.

- **Practice Deep Breathing**: Deep breathing helps activate the body's relaxation response, lowering heart rate and reducing feelings of anxiety. Try inhaling deeply for a count of four, holding your breath for four counts, and then exhaling slowly for four counts. Repeat this process a few times to help calm your mind and body.

- **Use Progressive Muscle Relaxation**: Progressive muscle relaxation involves tensing and relaxing each muscle group in your body, starting from your feet and working up to your head. This can relieve physical tension and help you feel more in control of your body during stressful situations.
- **Focus on the Present Moment**: Mindfulness encourages you to stay in the present moment rather than worrying about past or future events. If you start to feel overwhelmed, take a few moments to focus on your breathing, notice your surroundings, and ground yourself in the here and now. This can reduce stress and help prevent cognitive overload.

6. Pace Yourself Throughout the Event

Pacing yourself is essential for managing sensory overload during long or busy family gatherings. By balancing activity with rest, you can prevent fatigue from building up and reduce the likelihood of becoming overwhelmed.

- **Take Frequent Breaks**: Instead of waiting until you feel overwhelmed to take a break, incorporate regular rest periods throughout the event. This proactive approach can help you maintain your energy and prevent sensory overload before it starts.
- **Set a Time Limit**: Consider setting a time limit for how long you'll stay at the event. If a gathering is expected to last several hours, decide in advance how long you're comfortable staying. It's perfectly acceptable to leave early if you feel your energy levels dropping or if you start to feel overstimulated.
- **Prioritize Important Moments**: If the event includes several activities or interactions, prioritize the moments that are most important to you. For example, if you want to be present for dinner and gift exchanges, focus your energy on those parts of the event and take breaks during less essential activities.

7. Prepare for the Aftereffects of Sensory Overload

Even with the best strategies, it's possible that you may experience some degree of sensory overload during a family gathering. Preparing for the aftereffects can help you recover more quickly and minimize symptoms.

- **Plan for Recovery Time**: After the event, schedule time to rest and recover. This might include taking a nap, lying down in a quiet room, or spending time in a low-stimulation environment. Giving your brain and body time to recover from sensory overload can prevent lingering symptoms such as headaches or fatigue.
- **Hydrate and Nourish Your Body**: Dehydration and hunger can make sensory overload symptoms worse. Make sure to drink plenty of water and eat a nutritious meal after the event to help your body recover.
- **Use Calming Techniques**: If you feel anxious or overstimulated after the event, use calming techniques such as meditation, breathing exercises, or listening to calming music to help soothe your nervous system.

Conclusion

Dealing with overstimulation at family gatherings can be challenging for individuals with hydrocephalus, but with the right techniques, you can manage sensory overload effectively and still enjoy the event. By planning for breaks, using sensory management tools, practicing mindfulness, and pacing yourself, you can navigate the noise, lights, and activity of family gatherings without becoming overwhelmed.

It's important to remember that setting boundaries and taking care of your own needs are essential for maintaining your well-being. With these strategies in place, you can participate in family gatherings while protecting yourself from sensory overload and ensuring that you feel comfortable and supported throughout the event.

Chapter 15: Setting Boundaries with Family and Friends
How to Communicate Your Needs Without Feeling Guilty

For individuals with hydrocephalus, navigating social situations with family and friends can be both rewarding and challenging. Maintaining a healthy balance between social interaction and self-care is essential for managing your condition and overall well-being. However, setting boundaries with loved ones—whether regarding your physical limitations, need for rest, or how you manage your symptoms—can feel difficult, especially if you fear being misunderstood or judged. Guilt and the desire to meet others' expectations can make boundary-setting even more challenging.

In this chapter, we'll explore the importance of setting boundaries for managing hydrocephalus, provide strategies for effective communication with family and friends, and offer tips on how to advocate for your needs without feeling guilty. By learning how to establish healthy boundaries, you can protect your health, reduce stress, and maintain strong relationships with your loved ones.

Why Boundaries Are Essential for Individuals with Hydrocephalus

Living with hydrocephalus requires managing symptoms such as headaches, fatigue, cognitive difficulties, and sensitivity to sensory stimuli. Balancing your health needs with social obligations can be overwhelming, particularly when well-meaning family and friends don't fully understand the challenges you face. Setting boundaries helps you prioritize your health while still engaging with loved ones in a meaningful way.

Here are a few reasons why setting boundaries is critical for individuals with hydrocephalus:

1. Prevents Symptom Flare-Ups

Hydrocephalus symptoms can be triggered or worsened by stress, overstimulation, physical exertion, and lack of rest. Setting boundaries allows you to manage these triggers by limiting exposure to situations that may increase your intracranial pressure (ICP) or lead to fatigue. Without clear boundaries, you may feel pressured to participate in activities that can cause flare-ups, making it harder to manage your condition.

2. Reduces Emotional Stress

Social obligations, such as attending family gatherings or participating in group activities, can create emotional stress if you're concerned about how your health needs will be perceived. Setting boundaries helps reduce this emotional burden by establishing clear guidelines about what you can and cannot handle. This can alleviate anxiety and give you more control over your interactions with others.

3. Allows for Self-Care

Boundaries create space for self-care, which is essential for managing hydrocephalus. Whether it's taking time to rest, attending medical appointments, or managing your medication schedule, having boundaries in place ensures that you can prioritize your health without feeling guilty about stepping away from social situations.

4. Strengthens Relationships

While it may seem counterintuitive, setting boundaries can strengthen your relationships with family and friends. When you communicate your needs clearly, your loved ones are more likely to understand your limitations and respect your well-being. This leads to healthier, more supportive relationships based on mutual understanding and respect.

Overcoming the Guilt of Setting Boundaries

One of the biggest challenges to setting boundaries is overcoming the guilt that often accompanies it. You may worry about disappointing others, being seen as selfish, or letting your family down by not participating in every activity or gathering. However, it's important to remember that setting boundaries is not about rejecting your loved ones—it's about protecting your health and maintaining a balanced life.

Here are some tips to help you overcome the guilt associated with setting boundaries:

1. Recognize That Self-Care is Not Selfish

Caring for yourself is not selfish—it's essential for managing a chronic condition like hydrocephalus. By prioritizing your health, you are ensuring that you can continue to be present and engaged in your relationships. Remind yourself that self-care allows you to show up for your loved ones in the long term, rather than burning out from overcommitting in the short term.

2. Shift Your Perspective

Instead of viewing boundaries as a way of keeping people out, see them as a way of ensuring that your interactions with loved ones are positive and sustainable. Boundaries help you engage with others in a way that honors your needs and limits, preventing resentment or frustration from building up over time.

3. Understand That You Can't Control Others' Reactions

When setting boundaries, it's natural to worry about how others will react. Some family members or friends may not fully understand your health condition, and their initial response may be disappointment or confusion. It's important to remember that you can't control how others react, but you can control how you communicate your needs. Over time, most people will come to respect your boundaries, especially if they understand that your decisions are based on health needs.

4. Practice Self-Compassion

It's normal to feel guilty when you're unable to meet others' expectations, but practicing self-compassion can help you manage these feelings. Be kind to yourself and acknowledge that setting boundaries is a necessary part of managing your health. Remind yourself that you are doing the best you can, and that your well-being comes first.

How to Communicate Your Needs Effectively

Effective communication is the key to setting boundaries with family and friends. Being clear, direct, and compassionate in your communication helps avoid misunderstandings and ensures that your loved ones understand your limitations and needs.

Here are some strategies for communicating your boundaries effectively:

1. Be Clear and Specific

When setting boundaries, clarity is essential. Vague or indirect communication can lead to misunderstandings, leaving others unsure of what you need. Be specific about what you are asking for, and explain how certain activities or situations affect your health.

Example:

- Instead of saying, "I might need to leave early," try saying, "I will need to leave by 8 p.m. to avoid feeling too tired and to manage my symptoms."

Being specific helps others understand the boundary and gives them the opportunity to plan accordingly.

2. Use "I" Statements

Using "I" statements helps you express your needs without sounding accusatory or blaming others. This approach keeps the focus on your experience and feelings, rather than making the other person feel responsible for your boundaries.

Example:

- Instead of saying, "You always make things too loud and overwhelming," try saying, "I feel overwhelmed when there's too much noise, and I need to step away when that happens to manage my symptoms."

"I" statements help maintain a positive tone and reduce the likelihood of defensiveness from the other person.

3. Explain the Reasoning Behind Your Boundaries

Providing context for your boundaries helps others understand why they are important. When people understand how your condition affects you and why you need certain accommodations, they are more likely to be supportive.

Example:

- "Because of my hydrocephalus, loud environments can cause headaches and fatigue, so I may need to take breaks or leave early if things get too noisy."

By explaining your reasoning, you are educating others about your condition and creating empathy, which can lead to better support from your loved ones.

4. Practice Assertiveness

Being assertive means confidently expressing your needs while respecting others. It's about finding a balance between advocating for yourself and maintaining healthy relationships. Assertiveness allows you to set boundaries without feeling guilty or aggressive.

Example:

- If a family member pushes you to stay longer at a gathering than you're comfortable with, you can respond assertively by saying, "I understand that you want me to stay, but I need to leave now to take care of my health. I hope we can spend time together again soon."

Assertiveness involves being firm and clear while remaining polite and respectful.

5. Set Boundaries in Advance

Whenever possible, it's helpful to set boundaries before a situation arises. This allows your family and friends to understand your limitations before the event and reduces the likelihood of misunderstandings or last-minute conflicts.

Example:

- "I'm looking forward to the holiday gathering, but I wanted to let you know that I may need to take breaks throughout the evening. I'll find a quiet space if things get overwhelming, and I might need to leave early depending on how I'm feeling."

By setting expectations in advance, you reduce pressure on yourself during the event and give others time to adjust their plans.

6. Offer Alternatives

If you need to decline an invitation or limit your participation in an event, offering an alternative can help maintain relationships and show that you still want to be involved in a way that works for you.

Example:

- "I can't stay for the whole party, but I'd love to join for the first couple of hours and then catch up again later this week for lunch."

Offering an alternative demonstrates your desire to stay connected while honoring your boundaries.

Dealing with Resistance from Family and Friends

While many family members and friends will be understanding and supportive of your boundaries, some may have difficulty accepting them. Resistance can stem from a lack of understanding about your condition, unrealistic expectations, or their own emotional needs.

Here are some tips for dealing with resistance while maintaining your boundaries:

1. Stay Calm and Patient

If someone reacts negatively to your boundaries, try to remain calm and patient. It's natural for people to feel disappointed or confused when their expectations aren't met, but over time, most people will adjust. Use this as an opportunity to educate them about your needs and explain why the boundary is necessary.

2. Reiterate Your Boundaries

If someone continues to push against your boundaries, it's important to stand firm while reiterating your needs. Be polite but clear about what you can and cannot do.

Example:

- "I understand that you're disappointed, but I need to leave now to take care of my health. I appreciate your understanding, and I hope we can catch up again soon."

By calmly restating your boundaries, you reinforce their importance and remind others that your health comes first.

3. Seek Support from Allies

If certain family members or friends are resistant to your boundaries, seek support from those who do understand. Having allies who respect your needs can make a big difference in navigating difficult situations. They can help advocate for you and provide emotional support when needed.

4. Know When to Step Away

In some cases, if a family member or friend continually disrespects your boundaries, you may need to limit your interactions with them for your own well-being. While this can be difficult, prioritizing your health is essential. You can still maintain relationships while setting limits on how much time you spend with individuals who don't respect your needs.

Conclusion

Setting boundaries with family and friends is a crucial part of managing hydrocephalus and maintaining your health. While it can feel difficult to communicate your needs, especially when you fear disappointment or guilt, boundaries help protect your well-being, reduce stress, and foster healthier relationships. By being clear, assertive, and compassionate in your communication, you can advocate for yourself without feeling guilty or selfish.

Remember, setting boundaries is an act of self-care, and it allows you to be present for your loved ones in a way that respects both your health and your relationships. With time, practice, and support, setting boundaries can become a natural and empowering part of managing your condition.

Chapter 16: Finding Quiet Time in Busy Environments
Tips for Creating Moments of Calm During Chaotic Gatherings

Busy environments, such as holiday parties, family gatherings, or large social events, can be overwhelming, especially for individuals with hydrocephalus. The constant noise, bright lights, crowded spaces, and high energy levels can lead to sensory overload, headaches, fatigue, and stress. To manage these situations and protect your well-being, it's important to find quiet moments of calm, even in the midst of chaos.

This chapter will provide detailed strategies for creating peaceful spaces, taking breaks, and finding quiet time during busy gatherings. By incorporating these techniques, you can enjoy social events without becoming overwhelmed, ensuring that you maintain your health and energy throughout the experience.

The Importance of Quiet Time for Individuals with Hydrocephalus

For individuals with hydrocephalus, quiet time is essential for managing symptoms such as headaches, cognitive fatigue, and sensory overload. Overstimulation from noise, light, and activity can lead to increased intracranial pressure (ICP), which can exacerbate symptoms like headaches, dizziness, and nausea. Taking regular breaks to rest and reset can help regulate ICP, reduce stress, and allow you to re-engage in social situations without feeling drained.

Here are some key reasons why finding quiet time in busy environments is important:

1. Prevents Sensory Overload

Sensory overload occurs when the brain becomes overwhelmed by too much input from the surrounding environment, such as loud sounds, bright lights, and constant movement. For individuals with hydrocephalus, this can lead to cognitive fatigue, headaches, and difficulty concentrating. Regular quiet breaks help prevent sensory overload by giving the brain time to recover.

2. Reduces Stress and Anxiety

Busy social environments can be emotionally and mentally exhausting, especially if you're navigating multiple conversations, dealing with noise, or managing the expectations of others. Finding moments of calm allows you to reduce stress and anxiety, helping you feel more in control of your environment.

3. Improves Focus and Cognitive Function

Social events often involve extended periods of socializing, which can be mentally taxing. For individuals with hydrocephalus, cognitive fatigue can make it difficult to focus on conversations, process information, or respond to social cues. Taking quiet breaks allows your brain to recharge, improving your focus and cognitive function when you rejoin the gathering.

4. Protects Energy Levels

Busy environments can quickly deplete your energy, leaving you feeling physically and mentally drained. Finding moments of calm helps conserve energy by giving you a chance to rest, reset, and recharge. This allows you to participate in social events without feeling completely exhausted by the end.

Strategies for Finding Quiet Time in Busy Environments

Finding moments of calm in a chaotic environment may seem challenging, but with the right strategies, you can carve out peaceful breaks to help you manage sensory overload and fatigue. Here are some practical tips for creating quiet time during busy gatherings:

1. Identify a Quiet Space in Advance

One of the most effective ways to find quiet time during a busy event is to identify a designated quiet space ahead of time. This could be a quiet room, a secluded outdoor area, or even your car, depending on the location of the event. Knowing where you can go to take a break will give you peace of mind and make it easier to step away when needed.

- **Scout the Location**: If you're attending a gathering at someone's home, ask your host if there is a quiet room you can use to rest. In public spaces, look for areas such as a balcony, patio, or outdoor seating area where you can retreat for a few minutes of peace.
- **Set Up a Rest Area**: If you're hosting or attending an event at a familiar location, set up a rest area with comfortable seating, dim lighting, and calming decor. This space can serve as your personal sanctuary when you need a break from the noise and activity.

2. Plan Regular Breaks

Instead of waiting until you feel overwhelmed to take a break, plan regular intervals throughout the event to rest and reset. By scheduling breaks proactively, you can prevent sensory overload before it starts and maintain better control of your energy levels.

- **Set a Timer**: Use your phone or a smartwatch to set reminders for regular breaks. For example, you could plan to take a five-minute break every hour or step away after each significant part of the event (e.g., after dinner or between activities). This prevents you from becoming overstimulated without realizing it.
- **Use Breaks to Recharge**: During your breaks, focus on relaxing activities that help you recharge. This could include deep breathing exercises, stretching, or simply sitting in silence. Avoid using breaks to check your phone or engage in tasks that require mental effort, as this can prevent you from fully resting.

3. Practice Mindfulness and Deep Breathing

Mindfulness and deep breathing are powerful techniques for calming the mind and body, especially in busy environments. These practices can help you stay centered and focused, even when there's a lot of noise or activity around you.

- **Mindful Breathing**: Practice mindful breathing by focusing on each breath you take. Inhale slowly through your nose, hold the breath for a few seconds, and exhale slowly through your mouth. This helps activate the body's relaxation response, reducing stress and lowering your heart rate.

- **Grounding Techniques**: Grounding techniques help bring your attention back to the present moment and reduce feelings of anxiety or overstimulation. One simple grounding technique is the "5-4-3-2-1" method: identify five things you can see, four things you can touch, three things you can hear, two things you can smell, and one thing you can taste. This can help you regain focus when you feel overwhelmed.

4. Use Noise-Canceling Headphones or Earplugs

Noise is one of the most common triggers of sensory overload in busy environments. Using noise-canceling headphones or earplugs can help reduce the volume of background noise and create a more peaceful atmosphere for your brain.

- **Noise-Canceling Headphones**: If you're in a loud or crowded setting, such as a holiday party or family gathering, wearing noise-canceling headphones can help block out distracting sounds. You can use them to listen to calming music, white noise, or a guided meditation while you take a break.
- **Earplugs**: If you prefer a more discreet option, consider using earplugs to reduce noise levels. Earplugs can help you focus on conversations or activities without being overwhelmed by background noise.

5. Take Short Walks

If the environment becomes too chaotic or overwhelming, stepping outside for a short walk can provide immediate relief. Walking allows you to physically remove yourself from the noisy environment and gives your brain time to reset.

- **Walk in Nature**: If possible, take a walk in a natural setting, such as a garden, park, or backyard. Nature has a calming effect on the mind and body, and being surrounded by greenery can help reduce stress and anxiety.
- **Practice Walking Meditation**: Walking meditation involves focusing on each step you take, paying attention to how your body feels as you move. This mindful approach can help calm your mind and provide a sense of peace during busy events.

6. Limit Exposure to Stimulation

When attending a busy gathering, it's important to be mindful of how much sensory input you're exposed to. Limiting your exposure to bright lights, loud sounds, and crowded spaces can help prevent sensory overload.

- **Sit in a Quiet Corner**: If possible, position yourself in a quieter part of the room, away from the main source of noise or activity. For example, if there's music playing, choose a seat farther from the speakers or band. If you're in a large group, sit near the edges of the gathering rather than in the center of the action.

- **Dim the Lights**: Bright or flashing lights can contribute to visual overload. If you're hosting or attending a gathering at a familiar location, dim the lights or use soft, ambient lighting to create a more calming atmosphere.

7. Communicate Your Needs with Others

Don't be afraid to communicate your need for quiet time with family and friends. Most people will be understanding if you let them know that you need to take occasional breaks to manage your symptoms. Setting expectations in advance can reduce any pressure you might feel to constantly engage with the group.

- **Explain Your Needs**: Let your family and friends know that you may need to take breaks during the event to rest and prevent sensory overload. You can explain how hydrocephalus affects your ability to handle loud or busy environments and why quiet time is important for your health.
- **Set Boundaries**: If certain activities or environments are particularly overwhelming, don't hesitate to set boundaries. For example, if loud music or crowded spaces trigger sensory overload, let your host know that you'll need to step away or leave early if things become too stimulating.

8. Create a Calming Ritual

Establishing a calming ritual can help you find moments of peace in busy environments. This ritual can be as simple as drinking a cup of herbal tea, taking a few deep breaths, or listening to soothing music. Having a go-to routine that helps you relax can make it easier to find calm, even in the midst of chaos.

- **Use Aromatherapy**: Aromatherapy can have a calming effect on the nervous system. Carry a small bottle of essential oil, such as lavender or eucalyptus, and use it during your breaks to help create a sense of calm. You can apply the oil to your wrists or temples, or simply inhale the scent for a few moments.
- **Practice Gentle Stretching**: Gentle stretching can relieve physical tension and help you feel more relaxed. During your breaks, take a few minutes to stretch your arms, neck, and shoulders. This can improve circulation and reduce feelings of fatigue.

Conclusion

Finding quiet time in busy environments is essential for individuals with hydrocephalus to manage sensory overload, reduce stress, and protect energy levels. By identifying quiet spaces, taking regular breaks, using mindfulness techniques, and communicating your needs with others, you can create moments of calm during even the most chaotic gatherings.

With these strategies in place, you'll be able to enjoy social events while maintaining your well-being and preventing symptom flare-ups. Ultimately, learning how to create peace amidst chaos allows you to participate fully in social gatherings while honoring your health and personal boundaries.

Chapter 17: Handling Holiday Stress on the Nervous System
Simple Relaxation Techniques and Breathing Exercises to Calm the Nervous System

The holiday season is a time for celebration, connection, and joy, but it can also bring heightened levels of stress. For individuals with hydrocephalus, managing stress is especially important because stress can exacerbate symptoms such as headaches, fatigue, and cognitive difficulties by affecting the nervous system and raising intracranial pressure (ICP). Learning to handle holiday stress with relaxation techniques and breathing exercises can help calm the nervous system, regulate ICP, and promote overall well-being.

In this chapter, we'll explore how holiday stress affects the nervous system, provide detailed relaxation techniques, and share simple breathing exercises that can help soothe the mind and body. By incorporating these strategies into your daily routine, you can navigate the holiday season with greater ease and reduce the impact of stress on your health.

The Impact of Holiday Stress on the Nervous System

Stress, whether emotional, physical, or mental, activates the body's "fight-or-flight" response—a survival mechanism that prepares the body to respond to perceived threats. This response is controlled by the sympathetic nervous system, which increases heart rate, raises blood pressure, and releases stress hormones such as cortisol. While the fight-or-flight response is helpful in short bursts, chronic or excessive stress can take a toll on the body, particularly the nervous system.

For individuals with hydrocephalus, stress can lead to increased intracranial pressure, triggering symptoms such as:

- **Headaches**: Stress can cause blood vessels in the brain to constrict, leading to tension headaches or migraines.
- **Fatigue**: The nervous system becomes overworked when constantly in a state of stress, leading to physical and mental exhaustion.
- **Cognitive Difficulties**: Stress can impair memory, concentration, and decision-making, which are already challenging for some individuals with hydrocephalus.
- **Emotional Distress**: The pressure to meet holiday expectations, attend social events, or manage family dynamics can create emotional stress, contributing to feelings of anxiety, frustration, or irritability.

Managing stress is critical for maintaining stable ICP and minimizing hydrocephalus symptoms during the holiday season. One of the most effective ways to handle stress is through relaxation techniques and breathing exercises that calm the nervous system.

How Relaxation Techniques Affect the Nervous System

Relaxation techniques work by activating the parasympathetic nervous system, which is responsible for the body's "rest-and-digest" response. This system helps counteract the effects of the sympathetic nervous system, reducing stress hormones, slowing the heart rate, and promoting feelings of calm. For individuals with hydrocephalus, activating the parasympathetic nervous system through relaxation techniques can help regulate ICP, reduce headaches, and improve emotional well-being.

Simple Relaxation Techniques to Calm the Nervous System

Here are several relaxation techniques you can incorporate into your daily routine to help manage holiday stress and calm the nervous system:

1. Progressive Muscle Relaxation (PMR)

Progressive muscle relaxation (PMR) is a technique that involves tensing and relaxing each muscle group in the body to release physical tension and promote relaxation. By focusing on the body's physical sensations, PMR helps shift attention away from stressors and into the present moment.

How to Practice PMR:

- Find a quiet, comfortable space where you can sit or lie down.
- Starting with your feet, tense the muscles in your toes for 5-10 seconds, then relax them completely for 15-20 seconds. Notice the difference between the tension and relaxation.
- Move up your body, tensing and relaxing each muscle group—your calves, thighs, abdomen, chest, arms, hands, shoulders, neck, and face.
- As you release each muscle group, focus on how the relaxation feels and let go of any residual tension.
- After you've completed the exercise, sit quietly for a few moments, enjoying the feeling of relaxation.

PMR helps reduce physical tension caused by stress and promotes a sense of calm throughout the body.

2. Guided Imagery

Guided imagery is a relaxation technique that involves visualizing peaceful, calming scenes to help reduce stress and anxiety. By engaging the imagination, guided imagery helps shift the mind away from stressors and encourages relaxation.

How to Practice Guided Imagery:

- Find a quiet, comfortable space to sit or lie down.
- Close your eyes and take a few deep breaths to center yourself.
- Visualize a peaceful place where you feel calm and relaxed. This could be a beach, a forest, a mountain, or any location that brings you a sense of peace.

- Imagine yourself in this place—notice the sights, sounds, smells, and sensations around you. For example, if you're at the beach, imagine the sound of waves, the warmth of the sun on your skin, and the feeling of sand beneath your feet.
- Stay in this peaceful scene for 5-10 minutes, allowing your body and mind to relax.
- When you're ready, take a few deep breaths and slowly open your eyes, bringing the sense of calm with you.

Guided imagery is especially helpful for managing holiday stress, as it allows you to escape from the hustle and bustle of the season and focus on peaceful, soothing imagery.

3. Mindful Meditation

Mindful meditation involves focusing on the present moment without judgment, allowing thoughts and feelings to come and go without becoming attached to them. This practice helps reduce stress by promoting awareness and acceptance, which can prevent stress from escalating.

How to Practice Mindful Meditation:

- Find a quiet place to sit in a comfortable position.
- Close your eyes and bring your attention to your breath. Notice the sensation of the breath as it enters and leaves your body.
- If your mind begins to wander, gently bring your focus back to your breath without judgment.
- Continue to observe your breath for 5-10 minutes, allowing thoughts to pass through your mind without attaching to them.
- When you're ready, open your eyes and take a few deep breaths before returning to your day.

Mindful meditation can help you stay grounded during busy holiday gatherings and reduce the emotional impact of stress.

4. Yoga or Gentle Stretching

Yoga and gentle stretching help release physical tension in the body, improve circulation, and activate the parasympathetic nervous system. Stretching also helps improve flexibility and can reduce the physical discomfort that comes with prolonged periods of sitting or standing during holiday events.

How to Practice Gentle Stretching:

- Set aside 10-15 minutes for gentle stretching.
- Focus on slow, deliberate movements that stretch the major muscle groups, such as the neck, shoulders, arms, back, and legs.
- Incorporate deep breathing into each stretch, inhaling as you stretch and exhaling as you relax.
- Pay attention to how your body feels, and avoid any movements that cause discomfort or pain.

Yoga poses such as Child's Pose, Cat-Cow, and Seated Forward Bend are particularly effective for calming the nervous system and relieving stress.

Simple Breathing Exercises to Calm the Nervous System

Breathing exercises are one of the quickest and most effective ways to calm the nervous system, as they directly influence the body's relaxation response. By slowing down your breath and focusing on your breathing pattern, you can lower your heart rate, reduce stress hormones, and promote feelings of calm.

Here are some simple breathing exercises you can practice during the holiday season:

1. Diaphragmatic Breathing (Belly Breathing)

Diaphragmatic breathing, also known as belly breathing, involves breathing deeply into the diaphragm rather than shallowly into the chest. This type of breathing activates the parasympathetic nervous system, helping to reduce stress and promote relaxation.

How to Practice Diaphragmatic Breathing:

- Sit or lie down in a comfortable position.
- Place one hand on your chest and the other on your abdomen.
- Inhale deeply through your nose, allowing your abdomen to rise as you fill your lungs with air. Your chest should remain relatively still.
- Exhale slowly through your mouth, feeling your abdomen fall as you release the air.
- Continue this pattern for 5-10 minutes, focusing on the rise and fall of your abdomen with each breath.

Diaphragmatic breathing is an excellent tool for calming the nervous system during moments of heightened stress, such as holiday gatherings or busy family events.

2. 4-7-8 Breathing

The 4-7-8 breathing technique is a simple yet powerful exercise that helps regulate the breath and calm the nervous system. This exercise is particularly effective for reducing anxiety and promoting relaxation.

How to Practice 4-7-8 Breathing:

- Sit or lie down in a comfortable position.
- Inhale quietly through your nose for a count of 4.
- Hold your breath for a count of 7.
- Exhale completely through your mouth for a count of 8.
- Repeat this cycle for 4-8 breaths, focusing on the rhythm of your breathing.

The 4-7-8 technique slows down your breathing and helps bring your body into a state of relaxation.

3. Box Breathing (Square Breathing)

Box breathing, also known as square breathing, is a simple breathing technique that involves inhaling, holding, exhaling, and holding again for equal counts. This rhythmic breathing pattern helps regulate the nervous system and reduce stress.

How to Practice Box Breathing:

- Sit in a comfortable position with your feet flat on the floor.
- Inhale through your nose for a count of 4.
- Hold your breath for a count of 4.
- Exhale slowly through your mouth for a count of 4.
- Hold your breath again for a count of 4.
- Repeat this cycle for 5-10 minutes, focusing on the even rhythm of your breath.

Box breathing is particularly useful in high-stress situations, as it helps bring immediate relief by calming the mind and body.

4. Alternate Nostril Breathing

Alternate nostril breathing is a yogic breathing technique that helps balance the body's energy and promote a sense of calm. This exercise is effective for reducing stress and anxiety and can be especially helpful before or after a busy holiday event.

How to Practice Alternate Nostril Breathing:

- Sit comfortably with your spine straight and shoulders relaxed.
- Using your right thumb, close your right nostril.
- Inhale deeply through your left nostril.
- Close your left nostril with your right ring finger, and release your right nostril.
- Exhale slowly through your right nostril.
- Inhale through your right nostril, then close it with your thumb and release your left nostril.
- Exhale through your left nostril.
- Repeat this cycle for 5-10 breaths, focusing on the flow of air through each nostril.

Alternate nostril breathing helps bring a sense of balance and calm to the body, making it a useful tool for managing holiday stress.

Incorporating Relaxation and Breathing Exercises into Your Holiday Routine

To get the most benefit from relaxation and breathing exercises, it's important to incorporate them into your daily routine. Here are some tips for making these practices a regular part of your holiday season:

1. Start Your Day with Relaxation

Begin your day with 5-10 minutes of a relaxation technique, such as mindful meditation or deep breathing. This helps set a calm tone for the day and reduces the likelihood of stress building up throughout the day.

2. Take Breaks Throughout the Day

During the holiday season, it's easy to become overwhelmed by busy schedules, social events, and holiday preparations. Take short breaks throughout the day to practice a breathing exercise or engage in a relaxation technique. Even a few minutes of diaphragmatic breathing can help reset your nervous system and reduce stress.

3. Use Relaxation Techniques During Social Events

If you feel overwhelmed or stressed during a holiday gathering, use relaxation techniques or breathing exercises to calm your nervous system. You can step away to a quiet room for a few minutes to practice guided imagery or box breathing, or use diaphragmatic breathing while seated at the event.

4. End Your Day with Relaxation

Before going to bed, take 10-15 minutes to engage in a calming practice, such as progressive muscle relaxation or guided imagery. This helps prepare your body for restful sleep and reduces the effects of holiday stress on your nervous system.

Conclusion

The holiday season can be a time of increased stress, but with the right relaxation techniques and breathing exercises, you can calm your nervous system and protect your health. By incorporating practices such as diaphragmatic breathing, progressive muscle relaxation, and guided imagery into your daily routine, you can reduce the impact of stress on your hydrocephalus symptoms and maintain a sense of calm throughout the holiday season.

These simple yet effective techniques help regulate intracranial pressure, reduce tension, and promote emotional well-being, allowing you to navigate the holidays with greater ease and enjoyment.

Chapter 18: Managing Pain and Headaches

Strategies for Dealing with Increased Headaches and Discomfort During the Holidays

For individuals with hydrocephalus, headaches and discomfort can become more frequent or intense during the holiday season. The increased activity, stress, irregular routines, travel, and changes in diet can all contribute to heightened pain, particularly headaches that are often associated with fluctuations in intracranial pressure (ICP). Managing these symptoms requires a combination of proactive strategies, including stress reduction, pain management techniques, and healthy lifestyle choices.

This chapter will explore the causes of increased headaches and discomfort during the holidays and provide detailed strategies for preventing and managing these symptoms. By incorporating these techniques into your holiday routine, you can reduce the frequency and intensity of headaches and pain, allowing you to enjoy the season more fully.

Why Headaches and Discomfort Increase During the Holidays

For individuals with hydrocephalus, headaches are often linked to changes in intracranial pressure. Several factors that are common during the holiday season can contribute to fluctuations in ICP, leading to an increase in headaches, discomfort, and pain. Understanding the causes of these headaches is the first step toward managing them effectively.

Here are some of the most common triggers of headaches and discomfort during the holidays:

1. Stress and Anxiety

The holiday season often brings added stress due to social obligations, family gatherings, financial pressures, and holiday preparations. Stress activates the body's "fight-or-flight" response, releasing stress hormones such as cortisol, which can raise blood pressure and contribute to tension headaches or migraines. For individuals with hydrocephalus, stress can also lead to increased ICP, triggering headaches or worsening existing symptoms.

2. Changes in Routine and Sleep Patterns

Irregular routines, late nights, and disrupted sleep schedules are common during the holidays, especially with travel, parties, and family events. Sleep deprivation and inconsistent sleep patterns can lead to headaches, as the brain and body rely on regular rest to regulate ICP and repair themselves. Lack of sleep also increases sensitivity to pain, making headaches more intense.

3. Dehydration and Diet Changes

Holiday meals often involve rich, salty, and sugary foods, as well as alcohol and caffeinated beverages, all of which can contribute to dehydration. Dehydration is a major trigger for headaches, as it causes the brain to temporarily contract from fluid loss, leading to discomfort. Additionally, excessive sodium or sugar intake can raise blood pressure and lead to tension or migraine headaches.

4. Travel and Changes in Altitude

For individuals with hydrocephalus, long-distance travel—whether by car, train, or plane—can contribute to headaches due to prolonged periods of sitting, stress, and changes in altitude. Air travel, in particular, can lead to fluctuations in ICP due to cabin pressure changes, which can cause or worsen headaches. Additionally, dehydration caused by dry cabin air can intensify pain.

5. Overstimulation and Sensory Overload

Holiday events, especially large family gatherings, can involve loud noises, bright lights, and crowded spaces, all of which can trigger sensory overload. Overstimulation can cause headaches or migraines, especially for individuals with hydrocephalus, who may have heightened sensitivity to sensory input.

Strategies for Managing Headaches and Discomfort During the Holidays

Managing headaches and discomfort during the holiday season requires a proactive approach that addresses both the underlying triggers and the symptoms themselves. The following strategies can help you reduce the frequency and intensity of headaches and manage pain effectively:

1. Prioritize Stress Management

Since stress is a significant trigger for headaches, managing stress is essential for preventing pain during the holidays. By incorporating stress reduction techniques into your daily routine, you can help regulate your ICP and reduce the likelihood of tension headaches or migraines.

- **Practice Relaxation Techniques**: Techniques such as progressive muscle relaxation, guided imagery, and mindfulness meditation can help calm the nervous system and reduce stress. Regular practice of these techniques helps prevent headaches by promoting relaxation and reducing the impact of stress on your body.
- **Set Realistic Expectations**: The holidays often come with high expectations, both from yourself and others. To reduce stress, set realistic expectations about what you can handle, and don't be afraid to say no to commitments that feel overwhelming. Focus on activities that bring joy and avoid overloading your schedule.
- **Delegate Tasks**: If holiday preparations or social events are causing stress, delegate tasks to family members or friends. Sharing the responsibility can reduce your workload and prevent stress from building up.

2. Maintain a Consistent Sleep Schedule

Irregular sleep patterns and sleep deprivation are common during the holiday season, but maintaining a consistent sleep schedule is essential for preventing headaches. Sleep allows the brain to recover and regulate ICP, so getting enough rest is key to managing pain.

- **Stick to a Sleep Routine**: Try to go to bed and wake up at the same time each day, even on weekends or during holiday events. A regular sleep schedule helps regulate your body's internal clock and reduces the likelihood of sleep-related headaches.
- **Create a Restful Sleep Environment**: Ensure that your bedroom is conducive to restful sleep by keeping it dark, quiet, and cool. Use blackout curtains or an eye mask to block out light, and consider using earplugs or a white noise machine to minimize noise.
- **Avoid Screens Before Bed**: The blue light emitted by phones, tablets, and computers can interfere with your body's ability to produce melatonin, a hormone that promotes sleep. To improve your sleep quality, avoid using screens for at least an hour before bed.

3. Stay Hydrated

Dehydration is a common cause of headaches, especially during the holidays when rich foods, alcohol, and caffeine are more prevalent. Staying hydrated helps prevent headaches by maintaining the fluid balance in your body and brain.

- **Drink Water Regularly**: Aim to drink water throughout the day, especially if you're consuming salty foods, alcohol, or caffeine. Carry a refillable water bottle with you to remind yourself to stay hydrated.
- **Limit Alcohol and Caffeine**: Alcohol and caffeine are both diuretics, meaning they cause your body to lose more fluid through urine. To prevent dehydration, limit your intake of these beverages and alternate them with water. For every alcoholic or caffeinated drink, have a glass of water to maintain hydration.
- **Eat Water-Rich Foods**: In addition to drinking water, consume foods with high water content, such as fruits and vegetables. Foods like cucumbers, watermelon, oranges, and leafy greens help keep you hydrated and provide essential nutrients.

4. Manage Your Diet

Holiday meals are often rich, salty, and sugary, which can contribute to headaches by affecting blood pressure and hydration levels. Managing your diet by making healthier food choices can help prevent discomfort and pain.

- **Moderate Sodium Intake**: Foods high in sodium, such as processed meats, cheese, and salty snacks, can cause your body to retain fluids and raise blood pressure, leading to headaches. Try to moderate your intake of these foods and opt for low-sodium alternatives when possible.
- **Limit Sugary Foods**: While it's tempting to indulge in holiday treats, excessive sugar consumption can cause blood sugar spikes and crashes, which can lead to headaches. Enjoy sweets in moderation and balance them with healthier options like fruits or whole grains.
- **Eat Small, Frequent Meals**: Skipping meals or going too long without eating can cause blood sugar levels to drop, triggering headaches. To avoid this, eat small, frequent meals throughout the day to maintain stable blood sugar levels.

5. Take Breaks During Social Events

Large family gatherings, holiday parties, and busy environments can be overstimulating, leading to headaches or migraines. To manage sensory overload, take regular breaks during social events to rest and reset.

- **Step Away from Crowded Areas**: If the noise, lights, or activity at a social event become overwhelming, step away to a quieter space to give your brain time to recover. Find a quiet room, an outdoor space, or a less crowded area where you can take a break from the sensory input.

- **Use Noise-Canceling Headphones or Earplugs**: If loud noises are triggering your headaches, consider using noise-canceling headphones or earplugs to reduce the volume of background noise. These tools can help create a more peaceful environment and prevent sensory overload.
- **Practice Deep Breathing**: Deep breathing exercises can help calm your nervous system and reduce stress during social events. If you start to feel overwhelmed, take a few minutes to practice diaphragmatic breathing or box breathing to lower your heart rate and relax your mind.

6. Manage Travel-Related Headaches

Traveling during the holidays can trigger headaches due to changes in altitude, cabin pressure, dehydration, and stress. To manage travel-related headaches, plan ahead and take steps to minimize the impact of travel on your health.

- **Stay Hydrated During Travel**: Drink plenty of water before, during, and after your journey to prevent dehydration, especially if you're flying. Airplane cabins are notoriously dry, so bring a refillable water bottle and refill it regularly throughout the flight.
- **Manage Altitude Changes**: If you're flying or traveling to a high-altitude destination, be mindful of how altitude changes can affect your ICP. Use pressure-equalizing earplugs during takeoff and landing to reduce the impact of cabin pressure changes.
- **Take Breaks During Long Drives**: If you're traveling by car, take regular breaks to stretch, move around, and relieve tension. Sitting for long periods can lead to muscle stiffness and headaches, so it's important to get out of the car every hour or two for a short walk.

7. Use Pain Management Techniques

When headaches or pain do occur, it's important to have pain management techniques on hand to relieve discomfort and prevent symptoms from worsening. Here are some effective methods for managing headaches:

- **Apply a Cold Compress**: A cold compress applied to the forehead or back of the neck can help reduce headache pain by numbing the area and constricting blood vessels. Use a cold pack or wrap ice in a towel and apply it for 10-15 minutes at a time.
- **Take Pain Relievers**: Over-the-counter pain relievers, such as ibuprofen, acetaminophen, or aspirin, can help alleviate headache pain. Be sure to follow the dosage instructions and consult your healthcare provider if you have any concerns about using pain medication.
- **Practice Acupressure**: Acupressure involves applying pressure to specific points on the body to relieve pain. For headaches, applying pressure to the area between the thumb and index finger (known as the LI4 point) may help reduce discomfort. Use your opposite hand to press firmly on the point for a few minutes, then switch hands.

8. Monitor and Track Your Headaches

Keeping track of your headaches can help you identify triggers and patterns, allowing you to take preventive measures in the future. Use a headache diary to monitor when your headaches occur, what activities or foods may have triggered them, and how intense the pain is.

- **Record Headache Triggers**: Write down any factors that may have contributed to your headaches, such as stress, sleep patterns, diet, travel, or environmental changes. This information can help you make adjustments to prevent future headaches.
- **Note Pain Relief Methods**: Keep track of which pain management techniques are most effective for relieving your headaches. This can help you develop a personalized plan for managing pain when it occurs.

Conclusion

Managing headaches and discomfort during the holiday season requires a combination of preventive strategies and effective pain management techniques. By prioritizing stress reduction, staying hydrated, maintaining a consistent sleep schedule, and making mindful choices about diet and travel, you can reduce the frequency and intensity of headaches.

When headaches do occur, using pain relief methods such as cold compresses, deep breathing, and over-the-counter medications can help alleviate discomfort. By staying proactive and paying attention to your body's signals, you can navigate the holiday season with greater comfort and enjoy the festivities without being sidelined by pain.

Chapter 19: Temperature Control Indoors and Outdoors

Managing Your Environment to Prevent Cranial Pressure Fluctuations from Hot or Cold Weather

For individuals with hydrocephalus, temperature fluctuations—whether from hot or cold weather—can lead to cranial pressure changes, which may exacerbate symptoms such as headaches, dizziness, nausea, and fatigue. Both indoor and outdoor temperature changes can affect the body's ability to regulate intracranial pressure (ICP). Maintaining a stable and comfortable environment, especially during the extremes of summer heat or winter cold, is crucial for managing symptoms and ensuring overall well-being.

In this chapter, we will explore how temperature fluctuations affect individuals with hydrocephalus and provide detailed strategies for managing your environment both indoors and outdoors. By understanding the impact of temperature on your condition and learning how to create a more stable environment, you can prevent ICP fluctuations and reduce discomfort caused by weather changes.

How Temperature Affects Individuals with Hydrocephalus

The body relies on stable internal conditions to function optimally, and temperature regulation is a key part of this. For individuals with hydrocephalus, extreme temperatures—whether hot or cold—can disrupt the body's ability to regulate ICP, leading to symptom flare-ups. Here's how temperature fluctuations affect the body:

1. Heat and Increased Intracranial Pressure

Hot weather or high indoor temperatures can cause blood vessels in the brain to dilate, leading to an increase in blood flow to the brain. This increased blood flow can raise ICP, causing symptoms such as headaches, dizziness, and fatigue. Additionally, heat can lead to dehydration, which further exacerbates symptoms by reducing the amount of fluid available to regulate ICP.

- **Dehydration**: Hot weather causes the body to sweat more, leading to fluid loss. Dehydration reduces the volume of cerebrospinal fluid (CSF) in the brain, which can cause the brain to shift or increase ICP, triggering headaches.
- **Vasodilation**: Heat causes blood vessels to expand (vasodilation), which can lead to an increase in blood pressure within the brain, potentially raising ICP.

2. Cold Weather and Constricted Blood Vessels

Cold weather, on the other hand, causes blood vessels to constrict (vasoconstriction), which can reduce blood flow to the brain and lead to tension headaches or migraines. Cold environments may also cause the body to work harder to maintain its internal temperature, leading to fatigue and increased sensitivity to pain.

- **Vasoconstriction**: In cold weather, blood vessels narrow to preserve heat, which can reduce oxygen and nutrient delivery to the brain. This may lead to discomfort, headaches, or dizziness.
- **Muscle Tension**: Cold temperatures often cause muscle stiffness and tension, particularly in the neck and shoulders, which can contribute to tension headaches and increase discomfort.

3. Rapid Temperature Changes

Rapid changes in temperature—such as moving from a heated indoor environment to a cold outdoor setting—can cause the body to struggle to regulate ICP. These sudden shifts can trigger headaches, dizziness, or fatigue, making it important to avoid abrupt temperature transitions whenever possible.

Strategies for Managing Temperature Fluctuations Indoors

Indoor temperature control is essential for preventing cranial pressure fluctuations and ensuring comfort. Whether you're at home, at work, or visiting family during the holidays, creating a stable indoor environment can help reduce symptoms related to temperature changes.

1. Maintain a Comfortable Indoor Temperature

Keeping indoor temperatures consistent is key to preventing rapid changes in ICP. Aim for a temperature range that feels comfortable for your body, typically between 68°F and 72°F (20°C and 22°C). Avoid overheating your living space in winter or allowing it to become too warm in summer.

- **Use a Programmable Thermostat**: A programmable thermostat allows you to control the temperature in your home more efficiently, ensuring that your living environment remains stable throughout the day and night. Set the thermostat to maintain a comfortable temperature that avoids extremes of heat or cold.
- **Adjust Temperature Gradually**: If you need to raise or lower the temperature indoors, do so gradually to avoid sudden changes that can affect ICP. This can be particularly important when transitioning between rooms or adjusting the temperature for bedtime.

2. Use Fans or Air Conditioning in Hot Weather

In the summer or during warm indoor gatherings, it's important to keep cool to prevent overheating and dehydration. Using fans or air conditioning can help maintain a comfortable temperature and reduce the risk of cranial pressure fluctuations.

- **Fans**: Use ceiling or portable fans to circulate air and create a cooling effect, especially in areas where air conditioning may not be available. Make sure the airflow is directed in a way that provides relief without being too intense.
- **Air Conditioning**: If you live in a hot climate or are experiencing a heatwave, use air conditioning to keep indoor temperatures comfortable. Avoid setting the air conditioning too low, as this can cause sudden drops in temperature when moving from room to room.

3. Manage Humidity Levels

Humidity can significantly affect how hot or cold a room feels. High humidity in the summer can make the air feel warmer and cause excessive sweating, leading to dehydration. In winter, low humidity can cause dry air, which can contribute to sinus discomfort and headaches.

- **Dehumidifier**: In the summer or in areas with high humidity, use a dehumidifier to remove excess moisture from the air. This can help reduce the perceived heat and prevent dehydration.
- **Humidifier**: In winter or dry environments, a humidifier can add moisture to the air, preventing dryness that can exacerbate headaches and sinus pressure. Aim for a humidity level between 30% and 50% for optimal comfort.

4. Dress in Layers Indoors

Dressing in layers allows you to adjust your body temperature more easily, especially in environments where the indoor temperature may fluctuate due to heating systems or changes in activity levels (e.g., during holiday cooking or parties).

- **Wear Lightweight Layers**: In winter, wear lightweight, breathable layers that can be easily added or removed depending on the temperature. This allows you to stay warm without overheating.
- **Remove Layers if Overheating**: If you feel yourself becoming too warm indoors, remove outer layers and take a break in a cooler part of the room. Overheating can lead to dehydration, so be mindful of your body's signals.

5. Hydrate Regularly

Even indoors, it's easy to become dehydrated, especially in environments with heating or air conditioning. Staying hydrated helps regulate ICP and prevents headaches caused by dehydration.

- **Keep Water Accessible**: Always keep a bottle of water nearby, whether you're at home or visiting friends and family. Drink regularly throughout the day, especially if you're in a warm room or participating in holiday activities that may cause you to sweat.
- **Monitor Hydration Levels**: Pay attention to signs of dehydration, such as dry mouth, fatigue, or headaches. If you notice these symptoms, increase your water intake and take steps to cool down if you're feeling overheated.

Strategies for Managing Temperature Fluctuations Outdoors

When spending time outdoors, especially in extreme temperatures, it's important to take precautions to avoid triggering symptoms related to cranial pressure changes. Whether you're attending holiday festivities outside or simply running errands, here are some tips for managing temperature fluctuations in outdoor environments.

1. Dress Appropriately for the Weather

Dressing in weather-appropriate clothing is key to maintaining a stable body temperature and preventing discomfort or headaches caused by cold or heat.

- **In Cold Weather**: Wear warm, layered clothing in winter or cold conditions. Opt for a moisture-wicking base layer to keep sweat away from your skin, followed by insulating layers such as fleece or wool, and a waterproof outer layer if it's snowing or raining. Be sure to wear a hat or head covering to retain heat, but avoid hats that are too tight, as they can increase pressure on the head.
- **In Hot Weather**: In summer or hot environments, wear loose, lightweight clothing made of breathable fabrics such as cotton or linen. A wide-brimmed hat and sunglasses can help protect you from the sun's heat and reduce the risk of overheating. Be sure to wear sunscreen to prevent sunburn, which can exacerbate heat-related symptoms.

2. Take Breaks in the Shade or Indoors

If you're spending time outdoors in hot or cold weather, it's important to take regular breaks in a more comfortable environment. This helps prevent your body from becoming overwhelmed by extreme temperatures.

- **In Hot Weather**: Find shaded areas or air-conditioned spaces to take breaks and cool down. Sitting in direct sunlight for extended periods can lead to overheating and dehydration, both of which can increase ICP and trigger headaches.
- **In Cold Weather**: Step indoors periodically to warm up if you're outside in cold weather. Long exposure to cold temperatures can cause muscle tension, reduced circulation, and headaches, so it's important to give your body time to recover in a warmer environment.

3. Avoid Sudden Temperature Transitions

Sudden temperature changes, such as moving from a heated indoor space to the cold outdoors, can cause your body to struggle to regulate ICP, leading to headaches or discomfort. Whenever possible, transition gradually between temperature extremes.

- **Warm Up Slowly**: When entering a warm building after being outdoors in the cold, remove your outer layers gradually to avoid overheating. Give your body time to adjust to the warmer temperature without causing sudden shifts in ICP.

- **Cool Down Gradually**: In hot weather, avoid sudden exposure to cold environments such as air-conditioned buildings. Instead, cool down gradually by removing layers or resting in the shade before entering a colder space.

4. Monitor Physical Activity Levels

Engaging in physical activities, especially outdoors, can raise your body temperature and increase the risk of overheating. While physical activity is important for overall health, it's essential to manage your activity levels to avoid triggering headaches or cranial pressure fluctuations.

- **In Cold Weather**: While exercising in cold weather can help warm your body, be mindful of overexertion, which can cause you to overheat under layers of clothing. Adjust your pace and take breaks to avoid becoming too warm or too cold.
- **In Hot Weather**: Avoid intense physical activities during the hottest parts of the day, particularly in summer. If you do engage in outdoor activities, such as walking or light exercise, stay hydrated and take frequent breaks in the shade.

5. Use Cooling and Heating Accessories

Specialized accessories can help you maintain a stable body temperature when spending time outdoors, whether in hot or cold weather.

- **Cooling Accessories**: In hot weather, use cooling towels, neck wraps, or portable fans to keep your body temperature down. These accessories help regulate your temperature and prevent overheating, particularly if you're active outdoors.
- **Heating Accessories**: In cold weather, use hand warmers, heated gloves, or thermal socks to keep extremities warm. Additionally, heated blankets or seat warmers can be useful for staying warm when traveling by car or sitting outside.

Conclusion

Managing temperature fluctuations is crucial for individuals with hydrocephalus to prevent cranial pressure changes and related symptoms. Whether you're indoors or outdoors, maintaining a comfortable and stable environment helps reduce the risk of headaches, dizziness, and discomfort caused by extreme heat or cold.

By dressing appropriately, controlling indoor temperatures, staying hydrated, and avoiding sudden temperature transitions, you can better manage your environment and maintain your well-being during hot or cold weather. These strategies will allow you to enjoy the holiday season and other outdoor activities with greater comfort and fewer disruptions from temperature-related symptoms.

Chapter 20: Balancing Rest with Festivities
Finding a Healthy Balance Between Social Activities and Necessary Downtime

The holiday season is filled with social gatherings, family celebrations, and festive events that bring people together. For individuals with hydrocephalus, participating in these activities is often a joyful experience, but it can also be physically and mentally taxing. The increase in social obligations, changes in routine, and the demands of holiday preparations can lead to exhaustion, stress, and symptom flare-ups, such as headaches, fatigue, or cognitive difficulties.

Striking a balance between festive activities and necessary rest is essential for maintaining your health and well-being. In this chapter, we'll explore the importance of balancing social activities with downtime, provide practical strategies for managing your energy levels, and offer tips for communicating your needs to others. By finding this balance, you can enjoy the holiday season without overexerting yourself and causing unnecessary discomfort.

Why Balancing Rest and Social Activities is Important

For individuals with hydrocephalus, rest is not just a luxury—it's a necessity for managing symptoms and maintaining energy levels. Overexertion can lead to increased intracranial pressure (ICP), which can trigger headaches, fatigue, dizziness, and cognitive difficulties. These symptoms can worsen when you push yourself too hard during social events or holiday preparations without allowing enough time for recovery.

Here's why balancing rest with festivities is essential:

1. Prevents Symptom Flare-Ups

Social events often involve extended periods of activity, whether it's talking to family and friends, participating in holiday traditions, or traveling. These activities can be physically and mentally draining, especially when they occur back-to-back. Without adequate rest, the risk of symptom flare-ups—such as headaches, fatigue, and dizziness—increases.

2. Preserves Energy Levels

Festive gatherings and activities require both physical and mental energy. For individuals with hydrocephalus, energy levels may already be lower due to the condition's impact on the brain and body. Balancing rest with activities helps preserve your energy, allowing you to participate in important moments without feeling completely drained.

3. Reduces Stress and Overwhelm

The holiday season can be stressful, with its many social obligations, preparations, and expectations. Attending too many events without taking time to rest can lead to feelings of overwhelm, anxiety, or irritability. Incorporating downtime into your schedule helps reduce stress and allows you to manage social events with a clearer mind and calmer emotions.

4. Improves Cognitive Function

Cognitive fatigue is a common symptom of hydrocephalus, particularly after long periods of socializing or concentrating. Rest gives your brain the opportunity to recharge, improving your ability to focus, engage in conversations, and process information during social events.

Strategies for Balancing Rest and Festivities

Balancing rest with social activities requires careful planning, self-awareness, and the ability to prioritize your well-being. By using the following strategies, you can find a healthy balance between participating in holiday festivities and ensuring you get the rest you need to manage your symptoms.

1. Plan Your Schedule in Advance

One of the best ways to balance rest and festivities is to plan your schedule in advance. By knowing what events or gatherings you'll be attending, you can build in time for rest before, during, and after each event.

- **Review the Holiday Calendar**: Look at your holiday calendar to identify the major events and activities you plan to attend. Consider how much time each event will require, including travel time and preparation, and build in breaks between activities to allow for recovery.
- **Prioritize Key Events**: If your holiday schedule is packed with events, it's important to prioritize the ones that matter most to you. Focus on attending key events, such as family gatherings or holiday traditions, while giving yourself permission to skip or reduce participation in less important activities.
- **Avoid Overbooking**: Resist the temptation to pack your schedule with back-to-back events. Overbooking can quickly lead to exhaustion and symptom flare-ups. Instead, space out events by allowing for rest days between major gatherings.

2. Set Boundaries for Social Engagement

Setting boundaries is essential for balancing your energy levels and preventing social overload. Boundaries allow you to control how much time and energy you spend at social events, ensuring that you don't push yourself beyond your limits.

- **Limit the Duration of Events**: If you know that long events can be exhausting, set a time limit for how long you'll stay. For example, you can plan to attend a party for just two or three hours, rather than staying for the entire duration. Communicate your time limit to the host in advance so they understand why you may need to leave early.
- **Take Regular Breaks**: Even during social events, it's important to take regular breaks to rest and recharge. Step away from the main activity to find a quiet space where you can relax, take a few deep breaths, or engage in a calming activity. These short breaks help prevent sensory overload and reduce fatigue.
- **Say No When Necessary**: It's okay to decline invitations or opt out of certain events if you're feeling overwhelmed or fatigued. Saying no allows you to protect your energy and focus on the activities that are most meaningful to you. Remember that prioritizing your health is not selfish—it's essential for managing your condition.

3. Incorporate Rest into Your Daily Routine

Rest doesn't have to wait until after a social event. By incorporating rest into your daily routine, you can maintain a more balanced approach to holiday activities and reduce the likelihood of symptom flare-ups.

- **Schedule Downtime Each Day**: Set aside dedicated time for rest each day, whether it's taking a short nap, practicing relaxation techniques, or simply sitting quietly with a cup of tea. This helps prevent cumulative fatigue from building up over the course of the holiday season.
- **Use Rest Days to Recharge**: On days when you don't have any social events, focus on recharging by engaging in restful activities. This might include reading, meditating, watching a favorite movie, or taking a leisurely walk. These low-energy activities allow you to restore your physical and mental energy without putting extra strain on your body.
- **Practice Gentle Self-Care**: Self-care is an important part of maintaining balance during the holiday season. Gentle activities such as stretching, yoga, or deep breathing can help relax your body and reduce stress without requiring too much energy. Incorporating self-care into your daily routine ensures that you're taking care of yourself even amidst holiday busyness.

4. Manage Energy Levels with Nutrition and Hydration

The foods and drinks you consume during the holidays can have a significant impact on your energy levels and overall well-being. Maintaining a balanced diet and staying hydrated are essential for preventing energy crashes, headaches, and fatigue.

- **Eat Balanced Meals**: Focus on eating balanced meals that include a combination of protein, healthy fats, and complex carbohydrates. These nutrients help sustain your energy levels throughout the day, reducing the likelihood of fatigue during social events. Avoid heavy, sugary meals that can lead to blood sugar spikes and subsequent crashes.
- **Snack Wisely**: If you're attending a holiday event with rich or indulgent foods, snack wisely by choosing healthier options when possible. Opt for snacks that are high in fiber and protein, such as nuts, fruits, or whole grains, to maintain steady energy levels.
- **Stay Hydrated**: Dehydration is a common cause of headaches and fatigue, especially during the holiday season when alcohol, caffeine, and salty foods are more prevalent. Make sure to drink plenty of water throughout the day and during social events to prevent dehydration and keep your energy up.

5. Recognize Signs of Fatigue and Take Action

Listening to your body and recognizing the early signs of fatigue or symptom flare-ups is key to maintaining balance. By paying attention to how you feel during social events, you can take proactive steps to rest before your symptoms worsen.

- **Monitor Your Energy Levels**: Throughout the day or during social events, check in with yourself to assess how you're feeling. Are you starting to feel drained, overwhelmed, or lightheaded? If so, it's time to take a break, hydrate, or step away from the activity.
- **Identify Early Symptoms**: Headaches, dizziness, cognitive difficulties, and irritability are common signs that your body is becoming fatigued or overstimulated. Recognizing these symptoms early allows you to take action—whether by resting, eating, or hydrating—before the symptoms become more severe.
- **Respect Your Body's Limits**: It's important to respect your body's limits and not push through fatigue in the hopes of keeping up with social expectations. If you need to leave an event early, cancel plans, or take an extra day to recover, prioritize your health and do what's necessary to prevent symptom flare-ups.

6. Communicate Your Needs to Family and Friends

Family and friends may not always understand the need for rest or why you may need to take breaks during holiday gatherings. By communicating your needs clearly and assertively, you can set expectations and ensure that your loved ones support your efforts to balance rest with festivities.

- **Explain Your Condition**: If your family and friends aren't familiar with hydrocephalus and how it affects you, take the time to explain the condition and how certain activities can impact your energy levels. This helps them understand why rest is necessary and reduces any misunderstandings.
- **Be Clear About Boundaries**: When attending holiday gatherings, let your family and friends know if you'll need to take breaks, leave early, or limit your participation in certain activities. Being clear about your boundaries in advance helps set expectations and ensures that your loved ones can accommodate your needs.
- **Ask for Support**: Don't be afraid to ask for help or support when needed. Whether it's asking for a quiet space to rest during a family gathering or asking someone to take on a task you can't manage, leaning on your loved ones can help make the holiday season more enjoyable and less stressful.

7. Pace Yourself

Pacing yourself is one of the most effective ways to maintain a balance between social activities and rest. Rather than trying to fit everything into a short period, spread out your activities to give yourself time to rest and recover between events.

- **Space Out Activities**: If possible, schedule social events or holiday activities a few days apart to allow time for recovery in between. This prevents back-to-back events from overwhelming you and ensures that you can fully enjoy each gathering without feeling rushed or exhausted.
- **Take It One Day at a Time**: Focus on what you can manage each day, rather than trying to tackle everything at once. By pacing yourself and prioritizing what's most important, you can make steady progress without overexerting yourself.

Conclusion

Balancing rest with festivities is essential for individuals with hydrocephalus to manage energy levels, prevent symptom flare-ups, and reduce the physical and mental strain that often accompanies the holiday season. By planning your schedule in advance, setting boundaries, incorporating regular rest, and practicing self-care, you can find a healthy balance between participating in social activities and taking the downtime you need.

Ultimately, prioritizing your well-being and recognizing your limits allows you to enjoy the holiday season without overexerting yourself. By making thoughtful choices and pacing yourself, you can create a holiday experience that is both joyful and restful.

Chapter 21: Handling Last-Minute Holiday Changes
Coping with Spontaneous Plan Changes and Their Impact on Your Health

The holiday season is known for its joy and celebration, but it can also bring an element of unpredictability. Last-minute changes to plans—such as unexpected gatherings, shifting schedules, or sudden cancellations—are common during this time of year. While flexibility can be part of the holiday experience, for individuals with hydrocephalus, spontaneous changes can disrupt carefully planned routines and impact physical and mental well-being. Sudden adjustments can lead to stress, fatigue, and symptom flare-ups, making it essential to have strategies in place for managing these unpredictable moments.

This chapter will explore how last-minute holiday changes can affect your health and provide detailed coping strategies to help you stay calm, manage stress, and adapt to changes without compromising your well-being. By learning to navigate these situations effectively, you can minimize their impact and enjoy the holiday season with greater ease.

Why Last-Minute Changes Are Challenging for Individuals with Hydrocephalus

For individuals managing hydrocephalus, routine and structure are often important for maintaining a stable health condition. Disruptions to your schedule, such as spontaneous invitations or unexpected changes in plans, can lead to increased stress, fluctuations in intracranial pressure (ICP), and fatigue. Here's why last-minute changes can be particularly challenging:

1. Increased Stress Levels

Sudden changes to plans can trigger feelings of stress, particularly if they require you to rearrange your day or adjust to new expectations on short notice. Stress, in turn, can raise ICP and contribute to symptoms such as headaches, nausea, and dizziness. Additionally, the emotional stress of feeling unprepared or rushed can lead to anxiety, frustration, or irritability.

2. Disruption of Routine

Many individuals with hydrocephalus rely on consistent routines to manage their symptoms, including scheduled rest, medication, meals, and hydration. Last-minute changes can disrupt these routines, causing you to miss important rest periods or medication times, which can worsen symptoms or make it harder to recover from the stress of spontaneous events.

3. Difficulty in Managing Energy Levels

When plans change unexpectedly, it can be difficult to manage your energy levels, especially if the new plan requires you to engage in physical activity, social interaction, or travel that you weren't prepared for. This can lead to fatigue and overexertion, making it harder to participate fully in the new plan without feeling drained.

4. Overstimulation and Sensory Overload

Spontaneous changes in plans may expose you to environments or activities that cause sensory overload, such as loud gatherings, bright lights, or crowded spaces. Without time to prepare mentally or physically for these changes, sensory overload can quickly lead to headaches, discomfort, or cognitive fatigue.

Strategies for Coping with Last-Minute Holiday Changes

While last-minute changes are often unavoidable during the holiday season, you can take steps to minimize their impact on your health. The following strategies can help you stay flexible, manage stress, and adapt to sudden changes without compromising your well-being:

1. Stay Calm and Focus on What You Can Control

When faced with a last-minute change in plans, it's natural to feel stressed or overwhelmed. However, staying calm and focusing on what you can control can help you navigate the situation more effectively.

- **Pause Before Reacting**: When a spontaneous change occurs, take a moment to pause before reacting. This allows you to process the change and consider your options calmly, rather than rushing into a decision.
- **Break the Situation into Manageable Steps**: If the change feels overwhelming, break it down into manageable steps. For example, if you're invited to an unexpected event, focus on preparing for it one step at a time—choosing an outfit, organizing transportation, or packing necessary supplies—rather than becoming overwhelmed by the entire situation.
- **Focus on What's Within Your Control**: You may not be able to control the change itself, but you can control how you respond to it. Focus on the aspects of the situation that you can influence, such as how you prepare, when you arrive, or whether you choose to attend at all.

2. Communicate Your Needs and Boundaries

Effective communication is key to managing last-minute changes, especially when they affect your health and well-being. Being clear about your needs and boundaries helps others understand how the change may impact you and allows them to accommodate your situation.

- **Explain Your Condition**: If the last-minute change affects your ability to manage hydrocephalus symptoms—such as needing extra rest, avoiding overstimulation, or adjusting your medication schedule—explain this to your family or friends. This helps them understand why you may need to make modifications to the new plan.
- **Set Clear Boundaries**: If the spontaneous plan requires more energy than you have or conflicts with your need for rest, don't be afraid to set boundaries. For example, you can choose to attend part of the event but leave early if you start to feel fatigued. Be clear about your boundaries and communicate them to the host or organizer.
- **Say No When Necessary**: If a last-minute change feels too overwhelming or would significantly disrupt your health routine, it's okay to say no. Declining an invitation or opting out of a spontaneous event allows you to prioritize your health and avoid unnecessary stress. Remember that setting limits is a form of self-care, and your well-being comes first.

3. Adjust Your Schedule and Prioritize Rest

When last-minute changes disrupt your schedule, it's important to adjust your routine and prioritize rest to compensate for any disruptions. This ensures that you don't overextend yourself and that your body has time to recover.

- **Reschedule Rest Periods**: If a spontaneous change in plans affects your regular rest periods, make time for rest before or after the event. For example, if you need to attend a last-minute gathering in the evening, take a nap or relax in the afternoon to conserve energy for the event.
- **Prioritize Sleep**: Last-minute changes, such as late-night events, can affect your sleep schedule. If you need to attend an event that extends into the night, prioritize sleep afterward by going to bed earlier the next day or taking a longer rest period.
- **Plan for Recovery Time**: After spontaneous events, plan for recovery time to rest and recharge. This might include a quiet day at home, engaging in self-care activities, or avoiding social events for a day or two to allow your body to recuperate.

4. Pack an Emergency Kit for Spontaneous Events

Having an emergency kit on hand can help you manage symptoms if a last-minute change requires you to attend an unexpected event or travel on short notice. Your kit should include essential items that help you manage hydrocephalus symptoms and maintain your health routine.

- **Medication**: Always carry your medications, including pain relievers, in case you experience headaches or other symptoms while attending an event.
- **Hydration Supplies**: Bring a refillable water bottle to ensure you stay hydrated, especially if you're exposed to heat, alcohol, or rich foods that may contribute to dehydration.
- **Comfort Items**: Include items that help you stay comfortable, such as earplugs or noise-canceling headphones to block out loud noises, a hat or scarf to regulate body temperature, and a portable cold compress for headache relief.
- **Snacks**: Carry healthy snacks, such as nuts, fruit, or granola bars, to prevent blood sugar dips or provide energy during long events.

5. Use Relaxation and Breathing Techniques to Manage Stress

Last-minute changes can lead to feelings of stress, anxiety, or frustration, all of which can increase ICP and trigger symptoms. Using relaxation and breathing techniques can help calm your nervous system and reduce the impact of stress on your body.

- **Practice Deep Breathing**: Deep breathing helps activate the body's relaxation response, reducing stress and lowering your heart rate. Inhale deeply through your nose for four counts, hold for four counts, and exhale slowly through your mouth for four counts. Repeat this cycle until you feel calmer.

- **Use Mindfulness Techniques**: Mindfulness encourages you to focus on the present moment, helping you avoid becoming overwhelmed by the change. If you start to feel stressed, take a few moments to ground yourself by focusing on your breath or your surroundings.
- **Engage in Progressive Muscle Relaxation**: Progressive muscle relaxation involves tensing and relaxing each muscle group in your body, starting from your feet and working up to your head. This technique helps release physical tension caused by stress and can help you feel more relaxed before or during spontaneous events.

6. Prepare Mentally for Flexibility

Mental flexibility is key to handling spontaneous changes without becoming overwhelmed. By preparing yourself mentally for the possibility of last-minute changes, you can approach these situations with a more adaptable mindset.

- **Practice Accepting Change**: Accept that change is a natural part of life, especially during the holiday season, when plans can shift unexpectedly. By accepting that change may happen, you can approach these situations with less resistance and more flexibility.
- **Focus on the Positives**: Instead of focusing on the disruption, try to find positive aspects of the change. For example, a last-minute gathering might provide an opportunity to connect with loved ones or experience something new. Shifting your perspective can help reduce stress and make the change feel less overwhelming.
- **Be Kind to Yourself**: If last-minute changes cause stress or discomfort, be kind to yourself and recognize that it's okay to feel challenged by the situation. Practicing self-compassion can help you navigate the change without becoming overly critical or anxious.

7. Plan for Alternative Scenarios

Having a backup plan or alternative scenario in mind can help you feel more prepared when spontaneous changes occur. By anticipating potential challenges and preparing for different outcomes, you can approach last-minute changes with greater confidence.

- **Have a Backup Plan**: If you know that holiday plans may change, consider having a backup plan in place. For example, if a holiday gathering is moved to a different location, plan alternative transportation options or identify a quiet place where you can rest during the event.
- **Prepare for Early Exits**: If you're attending a spontaneous event, plan for the possibility of leaving early if the situation becomes overwhelming or if you feel fatigued. Make sure you have transportation options available and communicate your plan to the event host in advance.
- **Be Ready for Cancellations**: Sometimes, last-minute cancellations can be just as stressful as spontaneous invitations. If a holiday event is canceled, use the time for rest or engage in an activity that helps you recharge.

Conclusion

Last-minute holiday changes are inevitable, but they don't have to derail your health and well-being. By staying calm, communicating your needs, prioritizing rest, and using relaxation techniques, you can manage spontaneous changes without feeling overwhelmed. Having a flexible mindset and preparing for alternative scenarios also helps you stay adaptable and in control, ensuring that you can navigate the unpredictability of the holiday season with confidence.

Ultimately, balancing flexibility with self-care allows you to enjoy the holidays without compromising your health, giving you the tools to manage unexpected changes while protecting your energy and well-being.

Chapter 22: Hydrocephalus-Friendly Holiday Traditions
Adapting Old Traditions and Creating New Ones That Are Stress-Free

Holiday traditions are often at the heart of the season's joy, bringing families together and creating cherished memories. However, for individuals with hydrocephalus, participating in certain traditions can become overwhelming, especially when they involve high levels of activity, sensory stimulation, or stress. Adapting old traditions to suit your needs, or creating new ones that are more manageable, allows you to enjoy the season fully without compromising your health. This chapter explores how you can modify existing holiday traditions and introduce new ones that are hydrocephalus-friendly and stress-free, ensuring that you can take part in the festivities while prioritizing your well-being.

Why Adapting Holiday Traditions is Important

Traditional holiday activities, such as large family gatherings, elaborate meals, or traveling long distances, can place physical and mental strain on individuals with hydrocephalus. High levels of noise, crowded spaces, and the expectation to participate fully in every event can lead to sensory overload, headaches, fatigue, and increased intracranial pressure (ICP). By adapting traditions to accommodate your health needs, you can prevent symptom flare-ups and ensure that the holidays remain an enjoyable experience rather than a source of stress.

Here are some of the reasons why adapting holiday traditions is essential for individuals with hydrocephalus:

1. Reduces Physical and Mental Strain

Many holiday traditions involve activities that can be physically taxing, such as preparing large meals, decorating, or traveling to multiple locations. These activities can lead to fatigue and overexertion, especially if you're managing symptoms like headaches or dizziness. Adapting traditions to reduce physical strain helps ensure that you don't exhaust yourself or trigger a symptom flare-up.

2. Prevents Sensory Overload

Large gatherings, loud music, bright lights, and other sensory elements common during the holidays can lead to overstimulation and sensory overload. This is especially challenging for individuals with hydrocephalus, as overstimulation can increase ICP and cause headaches or cognitive fatigue. By modifying traditions to minimize sensory input, you can enjoy the holiday season in a more peaceful and controlled environment.

3. Allows for More Rest and Downtime

Traditional holiday activities often leave little room for rest, with packed schedules and long events that can stretch late into the night. This lack of downtime can make it difficult to manage symptoms effectively. Adapting traditions to include more opportunities for rest and relaxation ensures that you have the energy to participate without feeling drained or overwhelmed.

4. Encourages Inclusive Participation

By creating hydrocephalus-friendly traditions, you can ensure that everyone, including those with health challenges, can participate in the festivities. Adapting traditions allows you to involve all family members in ways that are enjoyable and manageable for everyone, fostering a sense of inclusion and connection.

Strategies for Adapting Old Holiday Traditions

Adapting old traditions doesn't mean giving up the activities you love—it's about finding ways to modify them so that they're more manageable and enjoyable for your current needs. The following strategies offer practical ways to adjust familiar holiday traditions while keeping the spirit of the season alive.

1. Simplify Holiday Gatherings

Large family gatherings are often a highlight of the holiday season, but they can also be overwhelming for individuals with hydrocephalus due to the noise, crowds, and extended social interactions. Simplifying these gatherings can make them more manageable and enjoyable.

- **Host Smaller, More Intimate Gatherings**: Instead of hosting or attending large gatherings with many guests, consider organizing smaller, more intimate get-togethers with a few close family members or friends. This reduces the sensory overload associated with large crowds and allows for more meaningful, low-stress interactions.
- **Limit the Duration of Events**: If holiday gatherings tend to stretch late into the night, consider shortening the event to a more manageable length. For example, hosting a holiday brunch or afternoon tea allows for festive socializing without the exhaustion of a long evening event.
- **Create Quiet Spaces**: If you're attending or hosting a holiday gathering, designate a quiet space where you can retreat if the noise or activity becomes overwhelming. This space should be free from loud music, bright lights, and heavy foot traffic, providing a peaceful place to rest.

2. Modify Traditional Holiday Meals

Preparing and hosting elaborate holiday meals can be a physically demanding and time-consuming task. If cooking large meals is stressful or tiring, consider simplifying your holiday dining traditions or sharing the responsibility with others.

- **Opt for Potluck-Style Meals**: Instead of preparing an entire meal by yourself, invite guests to contribute by bringing a dish. A potluck-style meal reduces the burden on the host while still allowing everyone to enjoy a variety of foods. You can focus on preparing one or two favorite dishes, while others handle the rest.
- **Simplify the Menu**: If you're used to preparing elaborate multi-course meals, simplify the menu to focus on a few key dishes that are easier to prepare and serve. Opt for recipes that require minimal preparation time or can be made in advance, reducing the pressure on the day of the event.

- **Host a Casual Holiday Gathering**: If the thought of preparing a traditional holiday dinner feels overwhelming, consider hosting a more casual gathering, such as a holiday brunch or dessert party. This allows for festive celebrations without the need for a formal, sit-down meal.

3. Adapt Travel Plans to Minimize Stress

For many families, traveling during the holidays is an important tradition, whether it's visiting relatives or going on vacation. However, travel can be stressful and physically demanding, especially if it involves long car rides, flights, or navigating crowded airports. Adapting your travel plans can help reduce the strain of holiday travel.

- **Consider Virtual Gatherings**: If travel is particularly stressful or difficult to manage, consider organizing virtual holiday gatherings using video calls. This allows you to stay connected with loved ones without the need for travel. You can even plan activities, such as a virtual holiday game night or gift exchange, to make the experience more festive.
- **Limit Long-Distance Travel**: If traveling long distances is unavoidable, plan your trip to minimize stress. This might include breaking up long car rides with frequent rest stops, traveling during off-peak times to avoid crowded airports, or choosing destinations that are closer to home.
- **Stay Close to Home**: Consider shifting your holiday tradition to focus on local events or celebrations that don't require extensive travel. Attending local holiday markets, light displays, or community events allows you to enjoy the season without the exhaustion of long-distance travel.

4. Adjust Holiday Decorating

Holiday decorating is a beloved tradition for many families, but it can also be physically demanding, particularly if it involves climbing ladders, lifting heavy boxes, or setting up elaborate displays. By simplifying your holiday decorating routine, you can still enjoy a festive atmosphere without the stress.

- **Focus on Key Areas**: Instead of decorating every room or covering your home in lights, focus on key areas that will create the biggest impact, such as the living room, entryway, or dining table. A few well-placed decorations can create a festive atmosphere without the need for extensive setup.
- **Use Simple and Easy-to-Manage Decorations**: Opt for decorations that are easy to set up and take down, such as string lights, garlands, or table centerpieces. Consider using pre-lit trees or wreaths that require minimal effort to assemble.
- **Involve Others in Decorating**: If decorating is an important tradition but feels overwhelming, enlist the help of family members or friends. Make decorating a group activity where everyone contributes, reducing the workload and making it a fun, shared experience.

Creating New, Hydrocephalus-Friendly Holiday Traditions

In addition to adapting old traditions, you can create new holiday traditions that are designed specifically to be low-stress, enjoyable, and manageable for your current needs. These traditions can still capture the festive spirit of the holidays while allowing you to participate fully without the physical or mental strain.

1. Create Relaxing Holiday Rituals

Incorporating relaxation and mindfulness into your holiday traditions can help reduce stress and promote a sense of calm during the season. These rituals allow you to connect with the holiday spirit without feeling overwhelmed.

- **Holiday Movie Night**: Host a cozy holiday movie night at home, complete with your favorite festive films, snacks, and comfortable seating. This tradition allows you to enjoy the holiday season from the comfort of your own home, without the need for travel or socializing in crowded spaces.
- **Mindful Holiday Activities**: Introduce calming holiday activities, such as baking holiday cookies, crafting homemade ornaments, or writing holiday cards. These activities provide a sense of accomplishment and festivity while promoting relaxation and creativity.
- **Evening Walks to View Holiday Lights**: If you enjoy holiday decorations but prefer a quieter, low-energy activity, consider taking evening walks to view holiday lights in your neighborhood. This simple tradition allows you to enjoy the beauty of the season while getting some fresh air and light exercise.

2. Incorporate Acts of Kindness and Giving

Focusing on acts of kindness and giving can be a meaningful way to celebrate the holidays, and it's a tradition that can be adapted to your energy levels and interests.

- **Volunteer from Home**: If you enjoy giving back during the holidays but find in-person volunteering too taxing, consider volunteering from home. This could involve making holiday cards for seniors, donating to a local food bank, or organizing a virtual fundraiser for a cause you care about.
- **Random Acts of Kindness**: Create a new tradition of performing random acts of kindness throughout the holiday season. These could include small gestures like paying for someone's coffee, donating warm clothes to a shelter, or leaving a kind note for a neighbor. This tradition focuses on the spirit of giving without requiring extensive time or energy.

3. Plan Low-Energy, Social Traditions

If you want to stay connected with loved ones during the holidays but need to avoid the exhaustion of large gatherings, consider creating new traditions that allow for social interaction in a more relaxed setting.

- **Holiday Book Exchange**: Organize a holiday book exchange with family or friends. Each person can choose a book they love or think others would enjoy and exchange it with someone else. This low-energy tradition allows for meaningful connection without the pressure of large social events.
- **Holiday Game Night**: Host a relaxed holiday game night with simple board games, card games, or trivia. This tradition can be done in person or virtually and provides an opportunity for fun and laughter without requiring too much physical or mental energy.
- **Holiday Puzzle Tradition**: Start a tradition of completing a holiday-themed puzzle as a family activity. Puzzles provide a quiet, engaging activity that encourages connection and conversation in a low-stress environment.

4. Focus on Quality Time Over Quantity

Instead of trying to attend every event or participate in every holiday tradition, focus on creating quality moments with loved ones. Meaningful, one-on-one interactions can often be more rewarding and less overwhelming than large, busy events.

- **Host a One-on-One Holiday Brunch**: Invite a close friend or family member for a relaxed, one-on-one holiday brunch. This allows for meaningful conversation in a calm, quiet setting, without the pressure of large social events.
- **Plan a Quiet Gift Exchange**: If gift-giving is an important part of your holiday traditions, plan a quiet, intimate gift exchange with a small group or one-on-one. This allows you to share the joy of giving without the stress of a large, noisy gathering.

Conclusion

The holidays are a time for connection, celebration, and joy, but they don't have to be overwhelming or stressful. By adapting old traditions and creating new, hydrocephalus-friendly ones, you can fully participate in the holiday season while prioritizing your health and well-being. Whether it's simplifying gatherings, introducing low-stress activities, or incorporating relaxation and mindfulness into your celebrations, finding traditions that work for you allows you to enjoy the holidays in a way that feels meaningful and manageable.

Ultimately, the most important part of the holiday season is the sense of connection and togetherness it brings. By creating traditions that honor your health needs, you can foster deeper connections with loved ones while making lasting memories in a way that supports your well-being.

Chapter 23: Gift Shopping with Ease
Managing Energy and Planning Shopping Trips to Avoid Stress

Gift shopping is one of the most anticipated—and often stressful—activities during the holiday season. For individuals with hydrocephalus, holiday shopping can be physically and mentally taxing, leading to fatigue, headaches, and sensory overload due to crowded stores, long lines, and the pressure to find the perfect gift. To make the experience more manageable and enjoyable, it's essential to plan your shopping trips carefully, manage your energy levels, and minimize stress.

This chapter provides strategies for navigating holiday gift shopping with ease, including how to plan and pace your trips, utilize online shopping options, and reduce sensory overload. By following these tips, you can enjoy the process of gift-giving without compromising your health or well-being.

Why Holiday Shopping Can Be Challenging for Individuals with Hydrocephalus

Holiday shopping requires both physical and mental effort, and for individuals with hydrocephalus, certain aspects of the experience can be particularly challenging. The following are common difficulties faced during holiday shopping:

1. Physical Fatigue

Shopping often involves long periods of walking, standing, carrying bags, and navigating crowded spaces. For individuals with hydrocephalus, these activities can lead to physical exhaustion, especially if fatigue is a common symptom of their condition. Prolonged physical exertion can also increase intracranial pressure (ICP), triggering headaches and other symptoms.

2. Sensory Overload

Holiday shopping environments—whether in malls or crowded stores—can be overwhelming, with bright lights, loud music, and large crowds. For individuals with hydrocephalus, these sensory stimuli can lead to sensory overload, which may cause dizziness, headaches, or cognitive fatigue. The constant need to process visual, auditory, and social input can become overwhelming, making shopping a draining experience.

3. Decision Fatigue

The holiday season often comes with the pressure to find the perfect gift for family and friends. Making numerous decisions about what to buy, comparing prices, and choosing between options can lead to decision fatigue, which can be particularly challenging for individuals who already experience cognitive difficulties due to hydrocephalus.

4. Time Pressure and Stress

The holiday shopping season can feel rushed, with limited time to find and purchase gifts. For individuals with hydrocephalus, the stress of feeling rushed or unprepared can lead to increased anxiety, which may exacerbate symptoms such as headaches, tension, and fatigue.

Strategies for Stress-Free Gift Shopping

Gift shopping doesn't have to be a source of stress. With careful planning and smart strategies, you can manage your energy levels, reduce sensory overload, and enjoy the process of selecting gifts for loved ones. Here are some key strategies to make holiday shopping more manageable:

1. Plan Your Shopping Trips in Advance

One of the best ways to minimize stress during holiday shopping is to plan your trips in advance. By creating a shopping plan, you can avoid feeling overwhelmed or rushed and ensure that your shopping experience is more organized and efficient.

- **Make a Shopping List**: Before heading out, create a detailed shopping list that includes all the gifts you need to purchase, as well as the stores or websites where you plan to buy them. Having a clear list helps you stay focused and reduces decision fatigue, as you won't need to browse aimlessly in stores.
- **Prioritize Gifts**: If your shopping list is long, prioritize the most important gifts first. This allows you to focus on the items that matter most and ensures that you have time to purchase them without feeling rushed. You can always return for less urgent items later.
- **Set a Budget**: Establish a budget for your gift shopping to avoid the stress of overspending. Knowing how much you're willing to spend on each gift makes it easier to narrow down your choices and prevents decision fatigue related to price comparisons.

2. Pace Yourself to Conserve Energy

Pacing yourself during holiday shopping is essential for avoiding physical exhaustion and managing your energy levels throughout the day. By breaking up your shopping trips into manageable chunks, you can prevent overexertion and ensure that you don't become too tired to enjoy the experience.

- **Break Shopping Into Smaller Trips**: Instead of trying to complete all your shopping in one day, break it up into smaller, shorter trips. For example, you can plan to visit two or three stores in one outing, then rest and return another day to visit the remaining stores. This allows you to conserve energy and reduces the risk of feeling overwhelmed.
- **Take Frequent Breaks**: During shopping trips, make a point to take regular breaks. Find a quiet place to sit, hydrate, and rest before continuing. This helps you avoid physical fatigue and provides a mental break from the sensory input of crowded stores.
- **Avoid Peak Shopping Times**: Shopping during peak hours, such as weekends or evenings, can increase the likelihood of dealing with large crowds and long lines, which can lead to stress and fatigue. Instead, try to shop during quieter times, such as weekday mornings or early afternoons, when stores are less busy and easier to navigate.

3. Utilize Online Shopping Options

Online shopping is a convenient way to purchase gifts without the physical and mental strain of visiting stores. Many retailers offer free shipping, gift wrapping, and even personalized gift options, making it easy to find thoughtful gifts from the comfort of your home.

- **Shop Online for Convenience**: Take advantage of online shopping to browse and buy gifts without leaving home. This allows you to avoid the physical demands of walking through stores and standing in lines, as well as the sensory overload of crowded shopping environments.
- **Use Wish Lists and Gift Guides**: Many online retailers offer wish lists and gift guides to help simplify the shopping process. You can browse curated selections of gifts based on price, interests, or recipients, which can reduce decision fatigue and make it easier to find the perfect present.
- **Compare Prices Online**: If you're unsure about where to find the best deals, use price comparison websites or apps to compare prices across different retailers. This allows you to shop efficiently and find the best value without spending time searching multiple stores.

4. Prepare for In-Store Shopping

If you prefer shopping in person, preparing for your outing in advance can help you manage your energy and prevent sensory overload. By planning ahead, you can create a more comfortable and stress-free shopping experience.

- **Wear Comfortable Clothing**: Dress in comfortable, breathable clothing that allows you to move freely and stay cool. Avoid heavy or tight-fitting clothes that could contribute to overheating or discomfort during long shopping trips.
- **Bring Essential Items**: Carry a small bag with essential items such as water, snacks, and any necessary medications. Staying hydrated and having a light snack on hand can help you maintain your energy levels, especially if you're shopping for an extended period.
- **Use Noise-Canceling Headphones or Earplugs**: If you're sensitive to loud environments, consider using noise-canceling headphones or earplugs while shopping. These tools can help block out overwhelming sounds and reduce sensory overload, making the shopping experience more manageable.
- **Ask for Help When Needed**: Don't hesitate to ask for assistance from store employees, especially if you need help finding specific items or have questions about products. This can save you time and energy while reducing the need to search through the store on your own.

5. Manage Decision Fatigue

The process of making decisions about gifts—such as choosing between products, comparing prices, and deciding what to buy for each recipient—can lead to decision fatigue. By simplifying your decision-making process, you can reduce mental exhaustion and make shopping more enjoyable.

- **Set Gift Categories**: Create gift categories for your recipients, such as "books," "kitchen gadgets," or "self-care items." This allows you to narrow down your options and focus on a specific type of gift for each person, reducing the overwhelming feeling of having too many choices.
- **Choose Simple, Thoughtful Gifts**: Focus on thoughtful but simple gifts that reflect the recipient's interests, rather than searching for elaborate or expensive items. A well-chosen book, candle, or personalized item can be just as meaningful as a more extravagant gift, without the stress of extensive decision-making.
- **Use Gift Cards**: If you're unsure what to buy for someone, consider giving a gift card to their favorite store or restaurant. Gift cards allow the recipient to choose what they want, taking the pressure off you to make the perfect choice.

6. Embrace Alternative Gift Ideas

Gift-giving doesn't always have to involve physical presents. If traditional gift shopping feels overwhelming, consider alternative gift ideas that are meaningful but less stressful to organize.

- **Give the Gift of Experiences**: Instead of buying physical gifts, consider giving the gift of experiences, such as tickets to a show, a museum pass, or a voucher for a special day out. Experiences are often more memorable and don't require you to navigate crowded stores or deal with wrapping and shipping.
- **Homemade Gifts**: If you enjoy creative activities, consider making homemade gifts such as baked goods, crafts, or DIY items. Homemade gifts are personal and thoughtful, and creating them can be a relaxing activity that allows you to focus on quality rather than quantity.
- **Donate in Someone's Name**: Consider donating to a charity in someone's name as a meaningful alternative to traditional gifts. Many organizations provide donation certificates or personalized acknowledgments, making this a thoughtful and stress-free option for gift-giving.

7. Practice Self-Care During Shopping Trips

Maintaining your physical and mental well-being during holiday shopping requires self-care. By focusing on your needs and recognizing when it's time to take a break, you can prevent shopping from becoming overwhelming.

- **Listen to Your Body**: Pay attention to your body's signals, such as fatigue, headaches, or dizziness, during shopping trips. If you start to feel tired or overwhelmed, take a break, sit down, or consider ending your shopping for the day. It's important to prioritize your health over completing your shopping list in one go.
- **Use Stress-Relief Techniques**: Practice stress-relief techniques such as deep breathing, progressive muscle relaxation, or mindfulness if you start to feel anxious or overstimulated. These techniques can help calm your nervous system and make the shopping experience more enjoyable.
- **Know When to Stop**: Don't feel pressured to finish all your shopping in one day or one trip. If you're feeling fatigued or overwhelmed, it's okay to stop and return another day. Taking care of yourself is more important than finishing your shopping on a tight timeline.

Conclusion

Holiday gift shopping can be a joyful experience when approached with a thoughtful plan and an emphasis on self-care. By managing your energy, pacing yourself, utilizing online shopping, and simplifying your decision-making process, you can reduce the physical and mental strain associated with holiday shopping. Whether you're browsing in stores or shopping online, these strategies will help ensure that gift shopping is a stress-free and enjoyable part of your holiday season.

Ultimately, the goal of gift shopping is to show your loved ones that you care. By approaching the process with a relaxed mindset and a focus on what matters most, you can make thoughtful gift choices without compromising your health or well-being.

Chapter 24: Choosing Safe, Comfortable Holiday Attire
Selecting Outfits That Won't Irritate or Affect Your Comfort

Dressing for holiday events and gatherings is an important part of the festive experience, but for individuals with hydrocephalus, it's essential to prioritize comfort alongside style. Certain clothing items—such as tight hats, scarves, or stiff fabrics—can increase discomfort by putting pressure on sensitive areas or restricting movement, which may lead to headaches, irritation, or fatigue. Choosing holiday attire that is both stylish and comfortable can help you enjoy the season's festivities without compromising your well-being.

In this chapter, we'll explore strategies for selecting comfortable holiday outfits that accommodate your health needs, including tips for choosing fabrics, avoiding tight accessories, and maintaining body temperature. By making thoughtful choices about your clothing, you can feel confident, comfortable, and ready to celebrate.

Why Comfortable Attire Is Important for Individuals with Hydrocephalus

Individuals with hydrocephalus often experience sensitivity in the head and neck area due to increased intracranial pressure (ICP) or the presence of a shunt. Wearing tight or restrictive clothing, especially around the head, can lead to discomfort or exacerbate symptoms such as headaches, pressure, or irritation. Additionally, holiday outfits are often worn for extended periods during long gatherings or events, so prioritizing comfort is essential for maintaining energy and preventing fatigue.

Here are some reasons why choosing comfortable holiday attire is crucial for individuals with hydrocephalus:

1. Reduces Pressure on the Head and Neck

Many traditional holiday accessories, such as hats, headbands, and scarves, can put pressure on sensitive areas around the head and neck, which can lead to discomfort or increase ICP. Individuals with hydrocephalus may experience headaches or pressure if these items are too tight or heavy.

2. Prevents Overheating or Chills

Temperature regulation is important for individuals with hydrocephalus, as extreme heat or cold can trigger symptom flare-ups. Overheating can lead to dehydration and increased ICP, while being too cold can cause muscle tension and discomfort. Choosing clothing that helps you maintain a stable body temperature is essential for staying comfortable during holiday events.

3. Maintains Comfort for Long Periods

Holiday gatherings often involve sitting or standing for long periods, making it important to choose clothing that allows for freedom of movement and doesn't cause irritation or discomfort.

Stiff fabrics, tight clothing, or heavy layers can become uncomfortable over time, leading to fatigue or soreness.

4. Supports Mobility and Flexibility

For individuals with hydrocephalus who experience mobility challenges or physical discomfort, it's important to choose clothing that supports ease of movement. Loose, flexible fabrics that allow for a full range of motion can help prevent strain and allow you to move comfortably throughout the event.

Strategies for Choosing Safe and Comfortable Holiday Attire

Selecting comfortable holiday attire requires a balance of style, functionality, and practicality. The following strategies will help you choose outfits that prioritize comfort without sacrificing your festive look:

1. Choose Soft, Breathable Fabrics

The fabric of your clothing plays a significant role in how comfortable you feel throughout the day or evening. Opting for soft, breathable fabrics helps prevent irritation and allows your skin to breathe, reducing the risk of overheating or feeling restricted.

- **Cotton and Linen**: These natural fabrics are lightweight, breathable, and soft against the skin, making them ideal for staying comfortable during indoor gatherings or warm environments. Cotton or linen shirts, blouses, and dresses can be both stylish and practical for holiday events.
- **Jersey Knit and Stretch Fabrics**: Jersey knit and fabrics with some stretch, such as cotton blends with elastane, provide flexibility and ease of movement. These fabrics are particularly comfortable for sitting or standing for long periods, as they won't dig into your skin or restrict motion.
- **Avoid Stiff or Scratchy Fabrics**: Fabrics like wool or sequins may look festive but can be scratchy or irritating, especially for individuals with sensitive skin. If you want to wear these materials, opt for pieces that are lined with a soft fabric, or wear a soft base layer underneath to prevent irritation.

2. Prioritize Loose, Non-Restrictive Clothing

Tight or restrictive clothing can increase pressure on the body, leading to discomfort and making it harder to move freely. Loose, non-restrictive clothing allows for better circulation, reduces pressure, and promotes comfort.

- **Flowing Dresses and Tunics**: Flowing dresses, tunics, or loose-fitting tops offer a stylish yet comfortable option for holiday events. These pieces allow for freedom of movement and won't cling tightly to your body, making them ideal for long gatherings.
- **Elastic Waistbands**: Pants or skirts with elastic waistbands provide more flexibility and are less likely to cause discomfort during extended wear. Look for stylish pants with an elasticized waist that maintains a polished look while offering comfort.

- **Layer with Loose Outerwear**: If you're attending an outdoor event or moving between indoor and outdoor spaces, opt for loose outerwear, such as an oversized coat or cardigan. This allows you to layer comfortably without feeling restricted by tight jackets or heavy coats.

3. Avoid Tight Hats, Scarves, and Headbands

Accessories like hats, scarves, and headbands are often worn during the holiday season, but they can cause discomfort if they're too tight or put pressure on sensitive areas around the head. Individuals with hydrocephalus, especially those with shunts, should be mindful of how these accessories fit.

- **Opt for Loose-Fitting Hats**: Choose hats that fit loosely around your head and don't press on your temples or forehead. Soft, stretchy knit hats or wide-brimmed hats made from flexible materials are good options. Avoid hats with tight bands or stiff structures that could cause pressure.
- **Use Lightweight Scarves**: If you need to wear a scarf for warmth, opt for a lightweight, soft fabric that drapes loosely around your neck. Heavy or tightly wrapped scarves can restrict movement and put pressure on your neck and shoulders, leading to discomfort. Infinity scarves made of light, breathable materials are a comfortable alternative.
- **Avoid Tight Headbands**: Headbands can add a festive touch to your holiday outfit, but they can also cause headaches if they're too tight. Opt for soft, elasticized headbands that sit gently on your head without squeezing. If possible, choose headbands with a wider band to distribute pressure more evenly.

4. Maintain Body Temperature with Layers

Temperature fluctuations during holiday events—whether from moving between indoor and outdoor spaces or from the heat of crowded gatherings—can lead to discomfort. Dressing in layers allows you to regulate your body temperature by adding or removing pieces as needed.

- **Wear a Base Layer**: Start with a soft, moisture-wicking base layer, such as a cotton or bamboo top, that can help regulate your body temperature. This layer should be breathable and comfortable against your skin, allowing you to stay cool if the event becomes warm or crowded.
- **Layer with a Light Sweater or Cardigan**: A light sweater or cardigan adds warmth without being too heavy. Look for pieces made from breathable fabrics like cashmere or cotton blends, which provide warmth without causing overheating. Cardigans are particularly convenient, as they can be easily removed if you start to feel too warm.
- **Choose Versatile Outerwear**: If you're attending outdoor events or traveling between locations, choose outerwear that is both warm and easy to layer over your outfit. A lightweight down jacket, puffer coat, or a stylish cape can provide warmth without being bulky. If the event is mostly indoors, opt for a light jacket that's easy to take off once inside.

5. Focus on Comfortable Footwear

Comfortable footwear is essential for navigating holiday events, especially if you'll be standing or walking for extended periods. Choose shoes that provide support, cushion your feet, and allow for easy movement.

- **Opt for Flats or Low Heels**: While high heels may be stylish, they can be uncomfortable and lead to foot pain or fatigue. Instead, choose flats, loafers, or low-heeled shoes that offer both comfort and style. Look for cushioned insoles and shoes with arch support to prevent foot pain.
- **Wear Boots with Cushioned Soles**: If you're attending an outdoor event or need to navigate cold, wet weather, opt for boots with cushioned soles and good arch support. Ankle boots or knee-high boots with a low heel provide both warmth and comfort, making them a great option for winter events.
- **Avoid Tight or Rigid Shoes**: Tight shoes or shoes made from rigid materials can cause discomfort, especially if you'll be wearing them for several hours. Choose shoes made from flexible, breathable materials that conform to your feet without squeezing or restricting them.

6. Choose Festive Yet Comfortable Accessories

Accessories are a great way to add a festive touch to your holiday outfit without sacrificing comfort. Look for accessories that are lightweight, soft, and easy to wear.

- **Opt for Lightweight Jewelry**: Heavy or bulky jewelry can become uncomfortable after a few hours, especially if it pulls on your ears or neck. Choose lightweight earrings, bracelets, and necklaces made from soft materials like leather, fabric, or delicate metals.
- **Use a Comfortable Bag**: If you're carrying a purse or bag to a holiday event, opt for one that is lightweight and easy to carry. Crossbody bags or small backpacks distribute weight more evenly, reducing strain on your shoulders or back. Avoid heavy, oversized bags that can lead to discomfort.

7. Dress for Flexibility and Mobility

If you experience mobility challenges due to hydrocephalus, it's important to choose clothing that allows for easy movement and doesn't restrict your range of motion.

- **Choose Stretchy Pants or Leggings**: Leggings or pants with stretchy, flexible fabrics provide comfort and mobility, allowing you to move freely without feeling restricted. Look for pants with an elastic waistband or pull-on style for added ease and comfort.
- **Opt for Wrap or Tunic-Style Tops**: Wrap tops or tunics offer a relaxed fit and easy movement, making them ideal for holiday gatherings where you'll be sitting, standing, or moving around. These styles are flattering and provide flexibility, allowing you to adjust them to your comfort level.

Conclusion

Choosing safe, comfortable holiday attire is essential for ensuring that you feel your best during festive events. By selecting soft, breathable fabrics, avoiding tight accessories, and layering for temperature control, you can maintain comfort while enjoying the season's celebrations. Prioritizing mobility and ease of movement allows you to participate fully in holiday activities without experiencing discomfort or fatigue.

Ultimately, your holiday attire should enhance your enjoyment of the season, allowing you to feel confident, stylish, and at ease. By making thoughtful choices about what you wear, you can celebrate the holidays comfortably while staying true to your personal style and health needs.

Chapter 25: Support Systems During the Holidays
Leaning on Support Networks and Involving Others in Managing Your Health

The holiday season is a time for celebration and connection, but for individuals with hydrocephalus, it can also be physically and emotionally demanding. Managing symptoms such as headaches, fatigue, and cognitive difficulties while navigating social obligations, travel, and holiday events can feel overwhelming. During this time, having a reliable support system in place—whether it's family, friends, healthcare providers, or online communities—can make a significant difference in maintaining your well-being and enjoying the festivities.

This chapter will explore the importance of leaning on support networks during the holidays and provide strategies for involving others in managing your health. By fostering communication, setting boundaries, and building a support team, you can navigate the holiday season with greater ease, ensuring that your physical and emotional needs are met while still participating in the celebrations.

Why Support Systems Are Essential During the Holidays

For individuals with hydrocephalus, the holiday season can bring unique challenges. The increased social engagements, travel, sensory stimuli, and deviations from daily routines can trigger symptom flare-ups and fatigue. A support system provides practical assistance, emotional comfort, and a sense of security, helping you manage your condition more effectively during this busy time of year.

Here are some key reasons why having a strong support network is crucial during the holiday season:

1. Helps Manage Physical and Emotional Strain

The holidays can be physically taxing, with long gatherings, travel, and preparations adding to daily routines. A support system can help alleviate this strain by assisting with tasks, offering emotional reassurance, and providing physical support when needed.

2. Reduces Stress and Overwhelm

The pressure to meet holiday expectations—whether through gift-giving, attending events, or hosting gatherings—can lead to stress and anxiety. Support systems provide a source of guidance and relief, helping to reduce feelings of overwhelm by offering assistance and encouragement.

3. Offers Practical Help with Daily Needs

Managing hydrocephalus often involves balancing medical appointments, medication schedules, and daily routines. During the holidays, when routines are disrupted, having someone who can remind you of these needs or step in to assist with transportation, errands, or meal preparation can prevent stress and ensure your health is properly managed.

4. Provides Emotional Comfort and Encouragement

The holidays can evoke a range of emotions, including joy, stress, and sometimes sadness or isolation. A strong support system offers emotional comfort, allowing you to express your feelings without judgment. They can provide encouragement during challenging moments and celebrate positive experiences with you, reinforcing the emotional bonds that make the holidays meaningful.

Building and Utilizing Your Support Network

Creating a robust support system involves reaching out to the people around you and communicating your needs clearly. Whether your network consists of family, friends, healthcare professionals, or online communities, knowing how to effectively lean on these sources of support can help you navigate the holiday season with confidence and peace of mind.

1. Identify Your Support Team

The first step in building a support system is identifying the individuals who can provide assistance, whether they're family members, friends, or healthcare professionals. Different people in your life may offer different forms of support, so it's important to understand who you can rely on for specific needs.

- **Family and Close Friends**: These individuals are often your primary source of emotional and practical support. They can help with day-to-day tasks, accompany you to events, and provide comfort during difficult moments. Identify family members or friends who understand your condition and are willing to step in when needed.
- **Healthcare Providers**: Your healthcare providers, including doctors, neurologists, and physical therapists, are key members of your support team. They can offer medical advice, adjust treatments as necessary during the holidays, and provide resources to help manage symptoms.
- **Support Groups**: Online or in-person support groups for individuals with hydrocephalus can be valuable sources of information and encouragement. Connecting with others who understand your experience can provide emotional validation and practical tips for managing your condition during the holidays.

2. Communicate Your Needs Clearly

Clear communication is essential for ensuring that your support network understands your needs and can provide the right assistance. By being open about your condition, your symptoms, and the challenges you face during the holiday season, you can set realistic expectations and ask for the help you need.

- **Be Specific About What You Need**: When reaching out to your support system, be clear and specific about what kind of help you're looking for. For example, you might ask a family member to help with holiday shopping, remind you to take medication, or assist with transportation to a medical appointment.
- **Explain Your Health Challenges**: If your family or friends aren't familiar with hydrocephalus, take the time to explain how the condition affects you, particularly during the holi-

day season. This can help them understand why you may need extra support, why you might need to take breaks during gatherings, or why certain activities may be challenging for you.

- **Set Boundaries**: Establishing boundaries is crucial for protecting your energy and managing symptoms. Communicate your limits to your support network—for example, if you need to leave an event early, take breaks, or opt out of certain activities. Clear boundaries prevent misunderstandings and help others respect your needs.

3. Involve Your Support Team in Holiday Planning

Involving your support system in the planning and execution of holiday activities can help reduce the physical and emotional burden on you, ensuring that you can enjoy the season without feeling overwhelmed.

- **Delegate Responsibilities**: Don't hesitate to delegate tasks to family or friends. If you're hosting a holiday gathering, for example, ask others to contribute by bringing food, helping with decorations, or setting up the event. This reduces your workload and allows you to focus on the aspects of the celebration that matter most to you.
- **Create a Backup Plan**: If you're attending a holiday event, communicate with a family member or friend who can step in if you start to feel fatigued or overwhelmed. They can help arrange transportation, guide you to a quiet space for rest, or assist with any unexpected needs that arise during the event.
- **Involve Healthcare Providers in Holiday Preparation**: If you anticipate challenges during the holiday season, schedule a check-in with your healthcare provider in advance. They can offer advice on managing symptoms during travel, attending gatherings, or dealing with last-minute changes in routine. Having a medical professional's input can provide peace of mind and help you plan for the holidays in a way that prioritizes your health.

4. Lean on Emotional Support

The holiday season can bring a mix of emotions, from joy and excitement to stress and even sadness. Having emotional support during this time is crucial for managing your mental well-being and preventing emotional strain from impacting your physical health.

- **Talk About Your Feelings**: Share your emotions with trusted family members or friends. Whether you're feeling joyful, stressed, or anxious, having someone to listen and validate your experiences can alleviate emotional tension. Opening up about how the holiday season affects you emotionally can also help prevent feelings of isolation.
- **Stay Connected to Support Groups**: Online or in-person support groups provide a safe space to connect with others who understand your unique challenges. Sharing your holiday experiences with others who have hydrocephalus can help you feel less alone and offer a source of mutual encouragement.
- **Practice Self-Compassion**: Be kind to yourself during the holiday season. It's normal to experience ups and downs, and it's important to acknowledge your efforts in managing your

condition. Practicing self-compassion helps prevent negative emotions like guilt or frustration from taking over, allowing you to focus on the positive aspects of the season.

5. Prepare for Travel and Events with Support

Travel and holiday events can be physically demanding and may require additional planning to ensure your comfort and safety. Lean on your support system to help manage the logistics of travel or prepare for holiday gatherings.

- **Travel with a Companion**: If you're traveling for the holidays, consider having a companion accompany you, whether it's a family member or friend. They can help with tasks like carrying luggage, navigating busy airports, or driving long distances. Having someone with you can reduce stress and provide practical assistance during the journey.
- **Coordinate Event Accessibility**: If you're attending a holiday gathering, work with the host to ensure the event is accessible and comfortable for you. This might include arranging for a quiet space to rest, ensuring that there's seating available, or requesting help with transportation. Involving your support system in these arrangements helps ensure that your health needs are met without adding unnecessary stress.
- **Use Technology to Stay Connected**: If you're unable to attend an event in person, consider using video calls or messaging apps to stay connected with loved ones. This allows you to participate in holiday celebrations remotely while still leaning on your support network for emotional comfort and connection.

6. Create a Supportive Holiday Environment

If you're hosting a holiday event or spending time at home during the holidays, creating a supportive environment can help reduce stress and make the season more enjoyable. Involve your support system in setting up an atmosphere that promotes relaxation, comfort, and joy.

- **Simplify Holiday Preparations**: Work with family members or friends to simplify holiday preparations. For example, you can reduce the number of decorations, opt for a potluck-style meal, or minimize the number of events you attend. A simplified holiday schedule allows you to focus on what matters most while reducing the physical and emotional strain of the season.
- **Designate Quiet Spaces**: Whether you're hosting or attending a holiday gathering, make sure there's a designated quiet space where you can retreat if you need a break. This space should be calm, comfortable, and free from noise or bright lights, providing you with a place to rest and recharge.
- **Foster a Positive Atmosphere**: Encourage family members and friends to create a positive, low-stress holiday atmosphere. This might include playing calming holiday music, dimming bright lights, and setting a relaxed tone for gatherings. A supportive and peaceful environment helps reduce sensory overload and allows you to enjoy the season without feeling overwhelmed.

Conclusion

The holiday season is a time for connection, celebration, and joy, but it can also bring challenges for individuals with hydrocephalus. Leaning on your support network—whether family, friends, healthcare providers, or online communities—can help you manage the physical and emotional demands of the season. By communicating your needs, setting boundaries, and involving your support system in holiday planning, you can ensure that your health and well-being are prioritized while still enjoying the festivities.

Ultimately, the key to a successful holiday season is not about doing everything on your own but rather about fostering a strong support system that helps you navigate challenges with ease. With the right support in place, you can approach the holiday season with confidence, knowing that you have a team of people who care about your well-being and are ready to help you enjoy the magic of the holidays.

Chapter 26: Children with Hydrocephalus: Parent Survival Tips
Helping Parents Support Children with Hydrocephalus During Holiday Activities

The holiday season is a time of joy and excitement, particularly for children, who look forward to holiday traditions, festive activities, and spending time with family and friends. However, for children with hydrocephalus, the busy pace of the season can sometimes be overwhelming or physically taxing. As a parent, it's important to provide the right balance of support and guidance to ensure that your child can participate in the holiday fun while managing their health and well-being.

In this chapter, we'll explore practical survival tips for parents of children with hydrocephalus. These tips focus on helping your child navigate holiday activities comfortably, managing symptoms, and creating an inclusive environment that allows your child to fully enjoy the magic of the season without becoming overwhelmed or fatigued.

Why the Holidays Can Be Challenging for Children with Hydrocephalus

Hydrocephalus affects the brain's ability to manage cerebrospinal fluid (CSF), and children with the condition often experience symptoms such as headaches, fatigue, and sensitivity to sensory stimuli. The holiday season, with its bright lights, loud music, crowded events, and increased physical activity, can exacerbate these symptoms. Additionally, changes in routine, travel, and new environments can make it harder for children to manage their health, leading to stress or discomfort.

Here are some specific reasons why holiday activities can be challenging for children with hydrocephalus:

1. Sensory Overload

Holiday events are often filled with bright lights, loud sounds, and lots of people, which can cause sensory overload for children with hydrocephalus. Sensory overload can lead to irritability, headaches, fatigue, and difficulty concentrating, making it harder for your child to enjoy the festivities.

2. Fatigue and Energy Management

Many holiday activities, such as parties, shopping trips, and family gatherings, require extended periods of physical activity or social interaction. For children with hydrocephalus, this can lead to fatigue, which may result in mood swings, difficulty engaging in activities, or even physical symptoms like headaches or dizziness.

3. Routine Disruption

Children with hydrocephalus often benefit from structured routines, including regular sleep schedules, medication times, and planned rest periods. The busy holiday season can disrupt these routines, making it harder for children to manage their symptoms and leading to potential health flare-ups.

4. Emotional Challenges

The excitement and pressure of the holiday season can lead to emotional ups and downs for any child, but children with hydrocephalus may be particularly sensitive to feelings of anxiety, frustration, or isolation. They may struggle with feeling different from their peers or siblings, especially if they are unable to participate fully in certain holiday activities due to their health.

Parent Survival Tips for Supporting Children with Hydrocephalus

As a parent, you play a crucial role in helping your child navigate the holiday season while maintaining their health and well-being. The following survival tips will help you provide the support, structure, and encouragement your child needs to enjoy holiday activities without becoming overwhelmed or fatigued.

1. Plan Holiday Activities with Your Child's Needs in Mind

The key to a successful holiday season is thoughtful planning that takes your child's health and energy levels into account. By being proactive, you can create a holiday schedule that includes fun activities while also allowing for rest and recovery.

- **Choose Age-Appropriate, Low-Stress Activities**: Focus on holiday activities that are manageable for your child's energy levels and physical abilities. For example, instead of attending large, crowded events, you can plan quieter activities like decorating cookies at home, watching holiday movies, or going for a drive to see holiday lights.
- **Create a Flexible Schedule**: While it's important to include fun activities in your holiday plans, build flexibility into the schedule to allow for rest breaks or adjustments based on how your child is feeling. Avoid back-to-back events, and leave room for downtime if your child becomes fatigued.
- **Limit the Number of Events**: Attending too many events can lead to sensory overload and fatigue. Prioritize the most important events or traditions, and consider skipping less critical activities. It's okay to say no to some invitations to ensure your child has enough energy for the experiences they enjoy most.

2. Manage Sensory Overload

Children with hydrocephalus may be more sensitive to sensory stimuli such as bright lights, loud music, and busy environments. Managing sensory overload is crucial for keeping your child comfortable and preventing irritability, headaches, or emotional meltdowns.

- **Choose Quiet, Low-Stimulation Environments**: When attending holiday events, try to find quieter spaces where your child can take breaks if they start to feel overwhelmed. For example, if you're at a family gathering, ask the host if there's a quiet room where your child can rest for a few minutes.
- **Use Sensory Tools**: Equip your child with sensory tools to help manage their environment. Noise-canceling headphones or earplugs can block out loud noises, while sunglasses or a hat with a brim can reduce the impact of bright lights. Weighted blankets or sensory fidget toys can also provide comfort during overstimulating situations.
- **Limit Screen Time**: While holiday movies and video games can be fun distractions, too much screen time can contribute to sensory overload. Encourage breaks from screens to prevent headaches and eye strain, especially after long periods of using electronics.

3. Pace Activities to Prevent Fatigue

Fatigue is a common challenge for children with hydrocephalus, and it's important to pace holiday activities to prevent overexertion. By scheduling regular breaks and balancing active and restful activities, you can help your child conserve energy and avoid symptom flare-ups.

- **Incorporate Rest Breaks**: Plan for regular rest breaks throughout the day, especially during long events or family gatherings. Allow your child to take short naps or quiet breaks in a peaceful room to recharge before returning to the festivities.
- **Alternate Between Active and Quiet Activities**: Balance high-energy activities like playing outside or attending a holiday event with quieter, more restful activities. For example, after an afternoon of holiday baking, your child could relax by reading a holiday book or doing a craft project.
- **Set Time Limits for Events**: If your child becomes tired easily, set a time limit for how long you'll stay at holiday events. Communicate this to family and friends in advance so they understand if you need to leave early or take breaks during the event.

4. Stick to a Routine When Possible

Maintaining a consistent routine can help children with hydrocephalus manage their symptoms and feel more secure during the busy holiday season. While some flexibility is necessary, try to stick to key elements of your child's routine, such as sleep schedules, medication times, and meal patterns.

- **Keep Bedtime Consistent**: While holiday events may sometimes extend into the evening, try to keep your child's bedtime as consistent as possible. Ensuring they get enough sleep each night will help prevent fatigue and improve their ability to handle holiday activities.
- **Stay on Track with Medication**: Make sure your child takes their medications on time, even when holiday schedules are busy. Set reminders on your phone or pack medications in advance if you're traveling or attending events.
- **Maintain Regular Meal and Snack Times**: Holiday gatherings often feature large meals and snacks, but it's important to maintain your child's regular eating schedule to prevent energy crashes. Pack healthy snacks and plan balanced meals to keep your child's energy levels steady throughout the day.

5. Support Emotional Well-Being

The excitement of the holiday season can sometimes bring emotional challenges for children with hydrocephalus, including feelings of frustration, anxiety, or isolation. Providing emotional support is essential for helping your child navigate the highs and lows of the season.

- **Validate Your Child's Feelings**: Encourage your child to express their emotions, whether they're excited, overwhelmed, or frustrated. Let them know that it's okay to feel a range of emotions during the holidays and that you're there to listen and support them.

- **Encourage Participation in Activities They Enjoy**: Help your child focus on the activities that bring them the most joy during the holiday season. Whether it's decorating, baking, or playing holiday games, encourage them to participate in ways that make them feel happy and included.
- **Foster Social Connections**: If your child is feeling isolated or different from their peers, help them stay connected with friends and family in ways that are comfortable for them. This could include virtual holiday calls with family, small playdates, or participating in online holiday events with friends.

6. Involve Your Child in Holiday Preparations

Allowing your child to be involved in holiday preparations can give them a sense of control and inclusion while also helping to keep activities manageable. Tailor the level of involvement to your child's abilities and energy levels.

- **Let Them Choose Activities**: Involve your child in choosing which holiday activities they'd like to participate in. This could include deciding which decorations to put up, selecting gifts for family members, or picking out a holiday movie to watch together.
- **Assign Simple Tasks**: Give your child age-appropriate tasks that make them feel included without overwhelming them. For example, they could help decorate cookies, set the table for a holiday meal, or wrap presents with assistance.
- **Create New, Low-Stress Traditions**: If traditional holiday activities feel too overwhelming, consider creating new, low-stress traditions that your child can participate in. For example, you could establish a family tradition of building a gingerbread house, crafting homemade ornaments, or taking a relaxing holiday walk around the neighborhood to see the lights.

7. Prepare for Travel with Support

Traveling during the holidays can be particularly challenging for children with hydrocephalus due to the physical demands of travel and the disruption of routine. If you're traveling, plan carefully to ensure your child's comfort and well-being throughout the journey.

- **Pack an Essentials Kit**: Prepare a travel kit with all of your child's necessary medications, snacks, sensory tools (such as noise-canceling headphones), and comfort items (such as a favorite blanket or stuffed toy). This ensures you have everything you need to manage symptoms and keep your child comfortable while on the go.
- **Plan for Rest Breaks**: If traveling by car, plan for regular stops where your child can stretch, rest, and take a break from the sensory stimulation of the journey. If flying, look for quiet areas in the airport where your child can rest between flights.
- **Stick to a Simplified Routine**: While it's important to be flexible during travel, try to stick to a simplified version of your child's routine as much as possible. Maintain regular meal times, ensure medication is taken on schedule, and prioritize sleep by bringing familiar sleep aids like a pillow or favorite bedtime story.

Conclusion

The holiday season can be a magical time for children, but for children with hydrocephalus, it's important to balance excitement with careful planning and support. By prioritizing your child's health, managing sensory overload, pacing activities, and maintaining routines, you can create a holiday experience that is both enjoyable and comfortable for your child.

As a parent, your guidance and support play a key role in helping your child navigate the season's challenges while still enjoying the joy and wonder of the holidays. By involving your child in holiday preparations, providing emotional encouragement, and creating a supportive environment, you can ensure that they experience the full magic of the holiday season in a way that feels manageable and fun.

Chapter 27: Handling Shunt Concerns Over the Holidays
What to Do if You Experience Shunt Malfunctions or Complications

For individuals with hydrocephalus, shunts play a critical role in regulating intracranial pressure (ICP) by draining excess cerebrospinal fluid (CSF) from the brain. While shunts are generally reliable, complications such as blockages, infections, or malfunctions can occur. Dealing with a potential shunt issue can be stressful at any time of year, but the holiday season—when travel, social obligations, and altered schedules are common—can make managing these concerns even more challenging.

This chapter provides detailed guidance on recognizing signs of shunt complications, preparing for potential issues during the holidays, and taking the right steps if a problem arises. By being proactive and prepared, you can navigate shunt-related concerns with greater confidence, ensuring your health and safety during the holiday season.

Common Shunt Complications and Symptoms

Shunt complications can range from mild issues to serious emergencies. Recognizing the early signs of a potential malfunction or infection is key to addressing the problem promptly. Below are some of the most common shunt-related complications and their symptoms:

1. Shunt Blockage or Obstruction

Shunt blockages occur when part of the shunt system becomes clogged, preventing proper drainage of cerebrospinal fluid. This can lead to a buildup of pressure in the brain, which can cause uncomfortable and potentially dangerous symptoms.

- **Symptoms of Shunt Blockage**:
    - Headaches (often intense and persistent)
    - Nausea and vomiting
    - Drowsiness or difficulty staying awake
    - Visual disturbances, such as blurred or double vision
    - Balance and coordination issues
    - Cognitive changes, such as confusion or memory problems
    - Swelling along the shunt tract (neck, abdomen, etc.)

If you or someone you care for experiences these symptoms, especially in combination, it could indicate a shunt blockage or malfunction. It's important to seek medical attention promptly.

2. Shunt Infection

Infections can occur in the shunt system, particularly after surgery or if there is a breach in the skin near the shunt. Shunt infections require immediate medical attention to prevent the infection from spreading to the brain.

- **Symptoms of Shunt Infection**:
    - Fever, chills, or sweats
    - Redness, warmth, or tenderness along the shunt tract
    - Swelling around the shunt area

- Irritability or unusual behavior changes (in children)
- Lethargy or drowsiness
- Nausea and vomiting
- Headaches or worsening hydrocephalus symptoms

Infections can escalate quickly, so it's important to recognize the signs and contact a healthcare professional immediately if these symptoms appear.

3. Overdrainage or Underdrainage

Shunt systems are designed to regulate CSF flow, but issues with overdrainage (removal of too much fluid) or underdrainage (removal of too little fluid) can occur. Both can lead to uncomfortable symptoms and may require medical intervention to adjust the shunt settings.

- **Symptoms of Overdrainage**:
  - Severe headaches, especially when standing or sitting upright (relieved when lying down)
  - Dizziness or lightheadedness
  - Nausea
  - Vision problems (blurred vision or difficulty focusing)
- **Symptoms of Underdrainage**:
  - Increasing headaches (similar to shunt blockage)
  - Nausea and vomiting
  - Irritability or behavioral changes (especially in children)
  - Drowsiness or difficulty waking up

Both overdrainage and underdrainage require adjustments to the shunt, so any of these symptoms should prompt a visit to a healthcare professional.

Preparing for Shunt-Related Concerns During the Holidays

The holiday season brings unique challenges—such as traveling, attending social events, and altered medical schedules—which can complicate the management of hydrocephalus and shunt care. Here are some proactive steps you can take to ensure you're prepared for potential shunt concerns during the holidays.

1. Keep Emergency Contact Information on Hand

Whether you're staying home or traveling during the holidays, it's important to have emergency contact information readily accessible in case of a shunt malfunction or complication.

- **Have Your Neurosurgeon's Contact Information**: Keep your neurosurgeon's or neurologist's contact information saved on your phone and written down in a place that's easy to access. This includes office numbers, emergency lines, and any direct contacts for urgent situations.
- **Locate Nearby Medical Facilities**: If you're traveling, research hospitals or medical facilities near your destination that are equipped to handle neurosurgical emergencies. Find out if they

have experience treating hydrocephalus or handling shunt complications, and save their contact details in case you need medical attention.

- **Communicate Your Condition to Others**: If you're attending a holiday gathering or traveling with family and friends, make sure at least one person knows about your condition and the signs of a shunt malfunction. This person should be familiar with how to respond in case of an emergency, including helping you seek medical attention.

2. Travel with Medical Records and Supplies

If you're traveling for the holidays, it's essential to bring your medical records, shunt information, and any necessary supplies to ensure you're prepared for potential issues. Having this information readily available can help healthcare providers treat you more effectively if an emergency arises.

- **Carry Shunt Documentation**: Travel with a copy of your shunt records, including the type of shunt you have, the valve settings, the manufacturer's details, and any past adjustments or surgeries. This information will be invaluable to doctors if a shunt complication occurs while you're away from your usual healthcare team.
- **Pack Essential Medications**: Ensure you have an adequate supply of any medications you regularly take to manage hydrocephalus symptoms, such as pain relievers or anti-nausea medications. Pack extra doses in case of travel delays or unexpected changes in plans.
- **Bring a Shunt Alert Card**: If you have a shunt alert card (often provided by your neurosurgeon), carry it with you at all times. This card contains important information about your shunt and can quickly inform healthcare professionals about your condition in an emergency.

3. Monitor Symptoms Closely

During the holidays, it's easy to become caught up in the excitement and overlook subtle symptoms that might indicate a shunt issue. However, it's important to stay vigilant and monitor your health closely.

- **Pay Attention to Early Warning Signs**: Headaches, nausea, fatigue, or changes in behavior are common early signs of a shunt malfunction. If you notice these symptoms, take action immediately—whether it's resting, reducing sensory stimulation, or contacting your doctor.
- **Don't Ignore Symptoms**: Even if you're in the middle of holiday festivities, don't dismiss symptoms. It's better to take a break or seek medical advice early than to risk a more serious issue developing.
- **Keep a Symptom Diary**: If you experience mild but persistent symptoms, consider keeping a diary to track any changes. This can help you identify patterns and provide your healthcare provider with detailed information if you need to schedule an appointment or call for advice.

What to Do if You Experience Shunt Malfunctions or Complications

If you or a loved one with hydrocephalus experiences symptoms of a shunt malfunction or complication during the holidays, it's essential to take action quickly. Here are the steps to follow if you suspect a shunt issue:

1. Stop and Rest

At the first sign of a possible shunt problem—such as a headache, nausea, or drowsiness—stop what you're doing and rest. Reducing sensory stimulation, sitting in a quiet environment, and lying down can help alleviate some symptoms, especially if they're related to overdrainage or sensory overload. However, rest alone may not be enough to resolve the issue, so proceed with the following steps.

2. Contact Your Healthcare Provider

If symptoms persist or worsen, contact your healthcare provider, even if it's outside of regular office hours. Most neurosurgeons and neurologists have an on-call system for emergencies, so you can speak to someone who can advise you on what to do next.

- **Describe Symptoms in Detail**: When speaking to your healthcare provider, describe your symptoms in detail. Mention when the symptoms started, how severe they are, and whether they've worsened over time. Provide any relevant context, such as recent travel, changes in routine, or physical activity.
- **Follow Their Advice**: Your healthcare provider will advise you on the next steps, which may include coming in for an evaluation, visiting an emergency room, or monitoring symptoms closely for further changes.

3. Seek Emergency Care if Necessary

If symptoms escalate quickly, or if your healthcare provider recommends immediate attention, seek emergency care right away. This is especially important if you experience severe headaches, vomiting, difficulty waking up, seizures, or any other signs of a serious shunt malfunction.

- **Go to the Nearest Emergency Room**: If you're traveling or away from your usual medical team, go to the nearest hospital with emergency care. If possible, choose a facility with neurosurgery services or experience in treating hydrocephalus. Bring your shunt records and medical documentation with you.
- **Advocate for Your Care**: In an emergency, you or a family member may need to advocate for your care. Ensure that medical staff are aware of your shunt and provide them with the necessary information about your condition. Don't hesitate to ask for a specialist if you believe the situation requires specific expertise.

4. Follow Up After an Emergency

If you experience a shunt-related emergency during the holidays, it's important to follow up with your neurosurgeon or neurologist as soon as possible after the event. Even if the issue was resolved in the emergency room, a follow-up appointment ensures that your shunt is functioning properly and that any necessary adjustments are made.

- **Schedule an Appointment**: Contact your healthcare provider after the emergency to schedule a follow-up evaluation. This may include imaging tests, such as a CT scan or MRI, to confirm that the shunt is functioning correctly.
- **Review Preventative Measures**: During your follow-up visit, discuss any preventative measures you can take to reduce the likelihood of future complications, especially if you experienced symptoms related to shunt overdrainage or underdrainage.

Conclusion

Shunt concerns during the holidays can be stressful, but with careful preparation and prompt action, you can manage potential complications effectively. By understanding the symptoms of shunt malfunctions, preparing for travel, and knowing when to seek medical attention, you can ensure your health and safety while still enjoying the holiday season.

Remember that staying vigilant, communicating with your healthcare team, and having a plan in place are key to handling shunt-related issues with confidence. The holiday season should be a time of joy and connection, and by being proactive, you can focus on celebrating while protecting your health.

Chapter 28: Holiday Event Safety Tips
Staying Safe at Holiday Parties, Parades, and Outdoor Events

The holiday season is filled with festivities, including parties, parades, and outdoor events that bring people together to celebrate. While these events can be joyous, they also come with certain risks, especially for individuals with hydrocephalus who may have heightened sensitivity to sensory stimuli, fatigue, or physical limitations. Ensuring your safety at these gatherings is essential for fully enjoying the holiday season without compromising your health or well-being.

This chapter provides detailed safety tips for attending holiday parties, parades, and outdoor events. By planning ahead, managing your energy levels, and taking precautions, you can participate in these celebrations while minimizing the risks associated with large crowds, environmental factors, and overstimulation.

Potential Safety Concerns at Holiday Events

Holiday events, while festive, often involve elements that can present challenges for individuals with hydrocephalus. Crowded spaces, loud noises, temperature extremes, and the potential for sensory overload are all factors that need to be considered when planning to attend these events. Recognizing the potential safety concerns in advance allows you to make informed decisions and take steps to protect your health.

Here are some common safety concerns you may encounter at holiday events:

1. Crowded Spaces

Holiday events such as parades, parties, and festivals often attract large crowds, which can create a variety of challenges. Navigating through crowds can be physically taxing, while the sheer number of people may lead to anxiety, sensory overload, or difficulty finding a quiet place to rest.

2. Sensory Overload

Many holiday events feature bright lights, loud music, and a high level of activity. These sensory elements can trigger headaches, dizziness, and fatigue for individuals with hydrocephalus, leading to discomfort or the need to leave the event early.

3. Temperature Extremes

Outdoor holiday events, such as parades, markets, or tree-lighting ceremonies, often take place in cold winter weather. Exposure to cold temperatures for long periods can increase the risk of muscle tension, shivering, and fatigue. On the other hand, indoor events can sometimes be overly warm, leading to overheating and dehydration.

4. Fatigue and Physical Strain

Attending long holiday events or parties that involve standing, walking, or socializing for extended periods can lead to physical fatigue. For individuals with hydrocephalus, fatigue can worsen symptoms such as headaches or dizziness, making it important to manage energy levels throughout the event.

5. Slips and Falls

Outdoor events, especially those held in winter conditions, can pose a risk of slips and falls due to snow, ice, or wet surfaces. Ensuring stability and minimizing the risk of injury is essential for staying safe at outdoor gatherings.

Safety Tips for Holiday Parties

Holiday parties are a staple of the season, whether they're small family gatherings or large social events. Attending these gatherings while managing hydrocephalus symptoms requires thoughtful planning and strategies to ensure your comfort and safety.

1. Choose Comfortable Seating and Take Breaks

If you'll be attending a party where seating is limited or standing is common (such as at a cocktail party), be mindful of how much time you spend on your feet. Long periods of standing can increase fatigue and discomfort, especially if you have mobility challenges or experience frequent headaches.

- **Find a Comfortable Seat Early**: Upon arrival, scope out seating options and choose a comfortable seat that allows you to take breaks throughout the event. If seating is limited, consider bringing a portable chair or cushion to ensure you have a place to rest when needed.
- **Take Regular Breaks**: Don't hesitate to take breaks during the party to rest in a quieter, less crowded area. These breaks help prevent sensory overload and give you time to recharge before rejoining the festivities.

2. Be Mindful of Noise Levels

Holiday parties can be noisy, with music, laughter, and conversations creating an environment that may be overwhelming for individuals with hydrocephalus. Managing noise levels is key to preventing headaches or discomfort caused by sensory overload.

- **Bring Noise-Canceling Headphones**: If you're sensitive to noise, consider bringing noise-canceling headphones or earplugs to help reduce the impact of loud environments. These tools allow you to enjoy the party while protecting your ears from overstimulation.
- **Seek Out Quieter Spaces**: Many large gatherings have quieter areas, such as a patio, balcony, or separate room, where you can escape the noise for a short time. Taking a break in a quieter space can help reset your energy levels and reduce the strain of constant auditory stimuli.

3. Stay Hydrated and Eat Mindfully

Holiday parties often feature rich foods and alcoholic beverages, which can contribute to dehydration, fatigue, and headaches. Staying hydrated and choosing your food carefully can help you manage your energy levels and avoid symptom flare-ups.

- **Drink Plenty of Water**: Make it a habit to drink water regularly throughout the event. If alcohol is being served, alternate between water and alcoholic drinks to prevent dehydration, which can exacerbate symptoms like headaches or dizziness.
- **Eat Balanced Meals**: Choose foods that provide sustained energy, such as those high in protein and fiber, rather than relying on sugary snacks or heavy meals. Eating balanced meals helps regulate blood sugar and prevents energy crashes later in the evening.

4. Communicate Your Needs to the Host

If you're attending a party hosted by family or friends, don't hesitate to communicate your needs in advance. Let the host know if you'll need certain accommodations, such as a quiet space to rest or assistance with transportation.

- **Request Accommodations**: If you know that certain aspects of the party environment (such as noise, lighting, or seating) may be difficult for you, discuss your concerns with the host ahead of time. Most hosts will be happy to make accommodations to ensure you're comfortable.
- **Arrange for Early Exits**: If the party extends late into the evening and you're concerned about fatigue, arrange for an early exit or set a time limit for how long you'll stay. Let the host know in advance that you may need to leave early to avoid feeling overextended.

Safety Tips for Holiday Parades and Outdoor Events

Outdoor holiday events, such as parades, festivals, and tree-lighting ceremonies, are a popular part of the season, but they also present unique safety challenges, especially when it comes to cold weather and large crowds. By taking the right precautions, you can enjoy these festive events while staying safe and comfortable.

1. Dress Warmly and Layer Appropriately

Outdoor events held in winter weather require careful attention to clothing. Cold temperatures, wind, and snow can lead to discomfort or even health risks if you're not properly dressed. Layering allows you to adjust your clothing based on changing temperatures or physical activity levels.

- **Wear Multiple Layers**: Start with a moisture-wicking base layer to keep sweat away from your skin, followed by insulating layers such as a fleece or wool sweater. Finish with a windproof and waterproof outer layer, such as a winter coat or parka, to protect against cold winds and precipitation.
- **Choose Comfortable Hats and Scarves**: Opt for soft, loose-fitting hats that don't put pressure on your head, especially if you have a shunt. Avoid overly tight scarves and choose materials that are both warm and comfortable, like cashmere or fleece.
- **Wear Warm, Non-Slip Footwear**: Winter weather often creates icy or slippery surfaces, so wear boots with good traction to prevent falls. Insulated boots will also help keep your feet warm during long outdoor events.

2. Bring Essential Supplies

Outdoor holiday events can last several hours, so it's important to bring supplies that will keep you comfortable and safe during the event.

- **Pack a Portable Seat**: If the event involves standing for long periods (such as a parade), consider bringing a foldable chair or portable seat. This allows you to sit and rest as needed, reducing the physical strain on your body.

- **Bring Snacks and Water**: Pack light, healthy snacks to maintain energy levels, especially if the event lasts several hours. Stay hydrated by bringing a water bottle, as dehydration can occur even in cold weather.
- **Carry Hand Warmers and a Blanket**: For extra warmth during cold outdoor events, bring hand warmers and a blanket. Hand warmers can help keep your hands toasty, while a blanket provides additional comfort during long periods of sitting.

3. Choose a Safe Viewing Spot

At outdoor events such as parades, choosing the right viewing spot can make a big difference in your overall safety and comfort. Avoid crowded areas and find a location that allows you to enjoy the event without being overwhelmed.

- **Avoid Crowded Areas**: Crowds can be overwhelming and make it difficult to find space to rest or move around. Look for a less crowded spot where you can sit comfortably and have a clear view of the event without being jostled by other attendees.
- **Stay Away from High-Traffic Zones**: If possible, avoid high-traffic zones such as entrances, exits, and pathways where people are constantly moving. These areas can become congested, making it harder to navigate and increasing the risk of falls or accidents.
- **Choose a Location with Shelter**: If the weather is unpredictable, try to find a spot near shelter, such as a covered area or building, where you can retreat if it starts to rain or snow. This provides a safe place to warm up if needed.

4. Be Aware of Your Surroundings

Staying aware of your surroundings is key to staying safe at crowded outdoor events, especially in large crowds or unfamiliar environments.

- **Keep an Eye on Exits**: Make note of the nearest exits and safe areas when you arrive. Knowing where to go in case of an emergency, or if you start feeling unwell, will help you leave the event quickly if necessary.
- **Stay with a Friend or Family Member**: It's always safer to attend large outdoor events with a companion. If possible, attend the event with a friend or family member who can help you navigate the crowd, carry belongings, or assist you if you start feeling fatigued or overwhelmed.
- **Avoid Hazardous Areas**: Be mindful of icy sidewalks, uneven terrain, or areas with poor lighting. If conditions are unsafe, choose a safer location or avoid the event altogether.

General Safety Tips for All Holiday Events

Whether you're attending a party, parade, or outdoor festival, these general safety tips will help ensure you stay safe and comfortable throughout the holiday season.

1. Listen to Your Body

Pay attention to how your body feels throughout the event. If you start to experience symptoms like headaches, dizziness, or fatigue, take action immediately—whether it's taking a break, finding a quieter space, or leaving the event.

2. Have a Plan for Early Exits

It's important to have a plan in place if you need to leave an event early due to discomfort or symptoms. Arrange for transportation ahead of time, and communicate with your friends or family about your intentions so they can support you if needed.

3. Stay Hydrated and Well-Nourished

Dehydration and hunger can exacerbate hydrocephalus symptoms, especially during long events. Drink water regularly, and eat balanced meals or snacks throughout the day to maintain your energy levels.

4. Take Breaks

Holiday events can be physically and mentally exhausting, so make sure to take regular breaks. Whether you're attending a party or a parade, taking short breaks will help you recharge and prevent sensory overload or fatigue.

Conclusion

Holiday events, whether they're parties, parades, or outdoor festivals, are an important part of the festive season, but they can also present challenges for individuals with hydrocephalus. By planning ahead, dressing appropriately, managing your energy levels, and taking safety precautions, you can enjoy these events while protecting your health and well-being.

Ultimately, the key to a successful holiday season is balancing fun with self-care. By making thoughtful choices and staying attuned to your body's needs, you can participate fully in the holiday celebrations and create lasting memories with friends and family.

Chapter 29: Dealing with Holiday Fatigue
Recognizing When to Step Back and How to Recharge During Extended Events

The holiday season is often filled with celebrations, social gatherings, and festive events that extend over several hours or even days. While these activities can be enjoyable, they can also lead to physical and emotional fatigue, especially for individuals with hydrocephalus. Managing energy levels is crucial to prevent symptom flare-ups, such as headaches, dizziness, and irritability, and to ensure that you can participate in the holiday season without becoming overwhelmed.

In this chapter, we'll explore how to recognize the signs of holiday fatigue and provide detailed strategies for stepping back, recharging, and maintaining your well-being during extended events. By understanding your limits and implementing self-care practices, you can balance holiday festivities with the rest your body needs to stay healthy and energized.

Understanding Holiday Fatigue

Holiday fatigue refers to the physical and emotional exhaustion that can result from the increased demands of the holiday season. For individuals with hydrocephalus, holiday fatigue may be exacerbated by the need to manage symptoms such as headaches, cognitive fatigue, and sensory overload. The busy schedule of holiday activities, combined with the pressure to attend social events, shop for gifts, and prepare for gatherings, can take a toll on your health if not managed carefully.

Common Causes of Holiday Fatigue:

1. **Overexertion**: Extended periods of physical activity, such as attending multiple events in one day, walking through crowded stores, or preparing large meals, can lead to physical fatigue and increased intracranial pressure (ICP).
2. **Sensory Overload**: Holiday environments are often filled with bright lights, loud music, and large crowds, which can overwhelm the senses and lead to headaches, irritability, and cognitive fatigue.
3. **Lack of Rest**: The busy pace of the holidays can make it difficult to prioritize rest, leading to sleep deprivation and exhaustion.
4. **Emotional Stress**: The holidays can bring emotional challenges, such as the pressure to meet social expectations or feelings of isolation. This emotional stress can contribute to mental and physical fatigue.

Recognizing the Signs of Holiday Fatigue

Recognizing the early signs of fatigue is essential for preventing burnout and allowing yourself time to recover before symptoms worsen. By paying attention to your body and mind, you can take proactive steps to step back and recharge before holiday fatigue takes a toll on your health.

Physical Signs of Holiday Fatigue:

- **Headaches**: Persistent or worsening headaches, especially after long periods of activity or socializing, may indicate that your body is becoming fatigued.

- **Muscle Tension**: Tension in the neck, shoulders, or back is a common sign of physical fatigue. This tension can be exacerbated by standing for long periods, carrying heavy items, or stress.
- **Dizziness or Lightheadedness**: Feeling dizzy, lightheaded, or unsteady can be a sign that you're overexerting yourself or not taking enough breaks.
- **Increased Sensitivity**: Heightened sensitivity to lights, sounds, or crowded spaces may indicate sensory overload and the need for a quieter environment.
- **Sleepiness or Drowsiness**: Struggling to stay awake or feeling unusually tired during the day is a clear sign that your body needs rest.

Emotional and Mental Signs of Holiday Fatigue:

- **Irritability**: Feeling irritable, short-tempered, or easily frustrated is a common emotional response to fatigue. You may find yourself less patient with others or less tolerant of stressful situations.
- **Difficulty Concentrating**: Cognitive fatigue can manifest as difficulty focusing, forgetfulness, or an inability to follow conversations. This may be particularly noticeable during social events or when trying to complete holiday tasks.
- **Mood Swings**: Rapid changes in mood, such as feeling overly emotional or anxious, can be a sign of mental exhaustion.
- **Overwhelm**: If you start to feel overwhelmed by your holiday schedule, social commitments, or the pressure to meet expectations, this is a sign that you may need to step back and prioritize self-care.

Strategies for Managing Holiday Fatigue

Once you recognize the signs of holiday fatigue, it's important to take action to prevent further exhaustion and recharge your energy levels. The following strategies will help you manage your energy, take necessary breaks, and maintain a healthy balance between participating in holiday events and caring for your health.

1. Prioritize Rest and Downtime

Rest is essential for preventing and managing holiday fatigue. Scheduling regular downtime and making rest a priority can help you recover from the physical and mental demands of the season.

- **Schedule Rest Periods**: Plan breaks throughout your day, especially during busy periods of holiday events. For example, if you're attending a party or shopping for gifts, set aside time before and after the event to rest and recharge.
- **Take Naps if Needed**: If you find yourself feeling fatigued during the day, don't hesitate to take a short nap to recharge. A 20- to 30-minute nap can help alleviate tiredness and improve focus.

• **Practice Good Sleep Hygiene**: Make sure you're getting enough sleep each night by maintaining a consistent sleep schedule and creating a relaxing bedtime routine. Avoid screens and stimulants before bed, and ensure your sleep environment is comfortable and quiet.

2. Set Boundaries and Limit Commitments

One of the main causes of holiday fatigue is overextending yourself by attending too many events or taking on too many responsibilities. Setting boundaries and limiting your commitments can help reduce the physical and emotional strain of the holiday season.

• **Be Selective About Events**: It's okay to say no to certain invitations or skip events that feel too overwhelming. Prioritize the gatherings that are most important to you, and don't feel guilty about opting out of others to protect your health.
• **Set Time Limits for Events**: If you're attending a long holiday event, such as a party or family gathering, set a time limit for how long you'll stay. Let the host know in advance if you plan to leave early so that you can manage your energy levels effectively.
• **Delegate Responsibilities**: If you're hosting a holiday gathering or involved in holiday preparations, delegate tasks to family members or friends. This reduces the burden on you and ensures that you have time to rest and recharge.

3. Take Breaks During Extended Events

Extended holiday events, such as long family gatherings or all-day shopping trips, can be exhausting if you don't take regular breaks. Incorporating short rest periods throughout the day can help you maintain your energy and prevent burnout.

• **Step Away for Quiet Time**: If you're feeling overwhelmed by a crowded or noisy environment, step away to a quieter area where you can rest. Take a few minutes to sit in a quiet room, go for a short walk outside, or simply close your eyes and take deep breaths.
• **Use Relaxation Techniques**: Practice relaxation techniques such as deep breathing, progressive muscle relaxation, or guided imagery to calm your mind and reduce stress. These techniques can be done in just a few minutes and are particularly helpful when you're feeling overstimulated.
• **Bring Comfort Items**: If you're attending a long event, bring comfort items such as a neck pillow, blanket, or noise-canceling headphones to help create a more relaxing environment when you take breaks.

4. Manage Sensory Overload

Holiday events are often filled with sensory stimuli, such as bright lights, loud music, and crowded spaces. Managing sensory overload is key to preventing fatigue and discomfort, especially during extended events.

- **Use Noise-Canceling Headphones**: If you're sensitive to noise, bring noise-canceling headphones or earplugs to block out loud sounds and create a more peaceful environment. You can wear them during busy parts of an event or when you need a break from sensory input.
- **Choose Quieter Environments**: Whenever possible, choose quieter areas to participate in holiday activities. For example, you might attend a smaller, more intimate gathering instead of a large party, or choose to sit in a quieter part of the room during a family dinner.
- **Limit Exposure to Bright Lights**: If bright holiday lights or flashing decorations are contributing to sensory overload, take breaks in dimly lit areas or wear sunglasses to reduce the impact of the lights. You can also position yourself away from brightly lit areas during indoor events.

5. Stay Hydrated and Eat Nutritious Foods

Proper hydration and nutrition are essential for maintaining energy levels and preventing fatigue. Holiday events often feature rich foods and alcoholic beverages, which can contribute to dehydration and energy crashes if not balanced with healthier choices.

- **Drink Water Regularly**: Stay hydrated by drinking water throughout the day, especially during long events. If alcohol is being served, alternate between alcoholic drinks and water to prevent dehydration, which can exacerbate symptoms like headaches or dizziness.
- **Eat Balanced Meals**: Choose foods that provide sustained energy, such as those high in protein, fiber, and healthy fats. Avoid relying on sugary snacks or heavy meals that can lead to energy crashes later in the day.
- **Bring Healthy Snacks**: If you're attending a long event or traveling during the holidays, bring healthy snacks such as nuts, fruit, or granola bars to maintain your energy levels and prevent hunger-induced fatigue.

6. Listen to Your Body

The most important strategy for managing holiday fatigue is to listen to your body and respond to its signals. If you start to feel tired, overstimulated, or unwell, take immediate action to rest and recharge.

- **Don't Push Through Fatigue**: If you start to feel fatigued during an event, don't try to push through it. Take a break, sit down, and rest until you feel ready to continue. Ignoring signs of fatigue can lead to more severe symptoms later on.

- **Give Yourself Permission to Leave Early**: If an event becomes too overwhelming or exhausting, it's okay to leave early. Your health and well-being should always come first, so don't feel obligated to stay longer than you're comfortable with.
- **Be Kind to Yourself**: It's easy to feel pressure to participate in every holiday event or meet every social expectation, but it's important to be kind to yourself and acknowledge your limits. Give yourself permission to rest, recharge, and focus on your health.

Conclusion

The holiday season is meant to be a time of joy and celebration, but it's also important to recognize when you need to step back and recharge. By being mindful of the signs of holiday fatigue, prioritizing rest, setting boundaries, and taking regular breaks during extended events, you can protect your health while still enjoying the festivities.

Ultimately, the key to navigating the holiday season with hydrocephalus is finding a balance between participation and self-care. By listening to your body and taking proactive steps to manage your energy levels, you can enjoy the magic of the holidays without becoming overwhelmed or fatigued.

Chapter 30: Explaining Hydrocephalus to Others

How to Explain Your Condition to Well-Meaning but Uninformed Family and Friends

For many individuals with hydrocephalus, the holiday season means spending time with family and friends who may not fully understand their condition. Hydrocephalus is a complex neurological condition, and explaining it to others—particularly those who are unfamiliar with its symptoms and effects—can feel challenging. Well-meaning family and friends may have questions, misconceptions, or assumptions about your health that make it difficult to communicate your needs clearly and comfortably.

In this chapter, we'll explore how to explain hydrocephalus to family and friends in a way that fosters understanding, support, and empathy. Whether you're addressing concerns about your energy levels, discussing the need for accommodations, or simply providing general information about the condition, these strategies will help you navigate conversations with loved ones so they can better support you during the holiday season and beyond.

Why Explaining Hydrocephalus Can Be Challenging

Hydrocephalus is not a condition that most people encounter on a daily basis, and as a result, family and friends may have little or no knowledge about it. They might not fully understand how the condition affects your daily life, or they may be unaware of the physical and emotional challenges you face. Some individuals might make assumptions about your capabilities or symptoms based on limited information, leading to misunderstandings or misconceptions.

Common challenges that arise when explaining hydrocephalus to others include:

1. Lack of Awareness

Many people are unfamiliar with hydrocephalus, and those who have heard of it may not understand the specifics of how it affects individuals. This lack of awareness can make it difficult for family and friends to grasp the nuances of the condition, leading to questions or misunderstandings.

2. Misconceptions About Symptoms

Some people may assume that because you don't "look sick," you don't experience symptoms. Hydrocephalus symptoms—such as headaches, cognitive difficulties, or fatigue—are often invisible, making it hard for others to recognize the severity of your condition.

3. Difficulty Discussing Medical Issues

Talking about personal health issues can be uncomfortable, especially if you're not sure how much detail to provide. You may worry about overwhelming others with too much information or feel uncertain about how to respond to well-intentioned but uninformed questions.

4. Concerns About Appearing "Different"

Some individuals with hydrocephalus may feel self-conscious about explaining their condition because they don't want to be treated differently or seen as "fragile." However, open communication is key to ensuring that your needs are met and that others can provide the right support.

Strategies for Explaining Hydrocephalus to Family and Friends

When explaining hydrocephalus to family and friends, it's important to strike a balance between providing enough information to foster understanding and keeping the conversation accessible and relatable. The goal is to help your loved ones understand how hydrocephalus affects you personally, so they can be supportive and empathetic.

1. Start with the Basics

Begin by explaining what hydrocephalus is in simple, straightforward terms. This gives your family and friends a basic understanding of the condition, providing context for the symptoms or challenges you may experience.

- **Definition of Hydrocephalus**: You can explain that hydrocephalus is a neurological condition in which excess cerebrospinal fluid (CSF) builds up in the brain, leading to increased pressure. This fluid buildup can cause a variety of symptoms, depending on the individual.
  - Example: *"Hydrocephalus is a condition where there's too much fluid in my brain, which increases pressure inside my head. The extra pressure can cause symptoms like headaches, fatigue, and dizziness."*
- **Mention the Role of a Shunt**: If you have a shunt (a device that helps drain excess fluid), explain its function briefly. This helps others understand how you manage the condition.
  - Example: *"I have a shunt, which is a small device that helps drain the extra fluid from my brain. It helps control the pressure, but it can malfunction sometimes, so I have to monitor my symptoms carefully."*

2. Describe How Hydrocephalus Affects You Personally

Hydrocephalus affects individuals in different ways, so it's important to explain how the condition impacts your daily life and specific holiday activities. Providing examples of your experiences helps others relate to your situation and understand the need for accommodations.

- **Explain Common Symptoms**: Share some of the common symptoms you experience, such as headaches, fatigue, or cognitive difficulties. Let your loved ones know that these symptoms can fluctuate and may be more pronounced during busy or stressful periods, such as the holidays.
  - Example: *"One of the main symptoms I deal with is headaches. They can be really intense, especially when there's a lot of noise or when I'm tired. That's why I might need to take breaks during family gatherings."*
- **Discuss Energy Levels**: If fatigue is a major challenge for you, explain how it affects your ability to participate in holiday events or activities. This helps others understand why you might need to limit your time at gatherings or take breaks to rest.
  - Example: *"I get tired more easily because of my condition, so I might need to leave the party early or step away for a rest. It's not that I don't want to be there—it's just that my energy levels can run low."*

- **Mention Sensory Sensitivity**: If you're sensitive to noise, bright lights, or crowded spaces, let your family and friends know so they can help create a more comfortable environment for you during events.
  - Example: *"I'm sensitive to loud sounds and bright lights because of the pressure in my head, so I might need to sit in a quieter space during the party. It helps me avoid getting overwhelmed."*

3. Be Honest About Your Needs

Openly discussing your needs is key to ensuring that you're supported during holiday events and gatherings. By being honest about your limitations and preferences, you can help others understand how they can accommodate you in a way that feels respectful and considerate.

- **Set Boundaries**: If certain activities or environments exacerbate your symptoms, communicate these boundaries clearly. Let your loved ones know that you may need to modify your participation to stay comfortable.
  - Example: *"I really enjoy spending time with everyone, but if the event gets too loud or crowded, I may need to take a break. I just want to make sure I'm taking care of my health while still being part of the celebration."*
- **Request Accommodations**: Don't hesitate to ask for specific accommodations that can make holiday events more comfortable for you. Whether it's access to a quiet room, extra seating, or flexibility with event timing, sharing your needs ensures that your family and friends can provide support.
  - Example: *"It would help if I could have a quiet room to rest in during the party if I start to feel tired. That way, I can recharge and still be part of the event."*
- **Ask for Understanding**: Let your loved ones know that while you may not be able to participate in every aspect of the holiday season, their understanding and support make a big difference.
  - Example: *"I may not be able to stay for the whole event, but I really appreciate your understanding. It means a lot to me to be included, even if I have to step back sometimes."*

4. Address Common Misconceptions

It's not uncommon for family and friends to have misconceptions about hydrocephalus, especially if they're unfamiliar with the condition. Addressing these misconceptions in a gentle and informative way helps correct misunderstandings and fosters a more supportive environment.

- **Clarify the Nature of the Condition**: Some people may assume that hydrocephalus is temporary or that it's something that can be easily "fixed." Gently explain that it's a lifelong condition that requires ongoing management.
  - Example: *"Hydrocephalus isn't something that goes away—it's something I manage every day. Even though I have a shunt, I still deal with symptoms, and there's always a risk of complications."*

- **Explain That Symptoms Can Be Unpredictable**: People may not realize that hydrocephalus symptoms can fluctuate based on factors like stress, physical activity, or sensory stimuli. Let them know that your symptoms may vary from day to day, and that it's important to listen to your body.
  - Example: *"Some days I feel pretty good, but other days I might have more headaches or fatigue. It really depends on what's going on, so I have to be flexible with my plans."*
- **Address the "You Don't Look Sick" Mentality**: If you've encountered the misconception that you don't "look sick" because your symptoms aren't always visible, explain that many aspects of hydrocephalus are invisible but still very real.
  - Example: *"Even though I might look fine on the outside, I still deal with a lot of symptoms that aren't always obvious, like headaches or dizziness. It's one of those conditions where you can't always see what's going on."*

5. Keep the Conversation Positive

While it's important to explain the challenges of living with hydrocephalus, it's also helpful to keep the conversation positive and focus on how your loved ones can support you. Reassure them that with the right accommodations, you can still participate in holiday activities and enjoy your time together.

- **Highlight What You Can Do**: While you may have certain limitations, emphasize the activities and events that you can enjoy. This helps shift the focus away from what you can't do and toward the ways you can still be involved.
  - Example: *"I might need to take breaks during the party, but I'm really looking forward to spending time with everyone and joining in on the gift exchange."*
- **Express Gratitude for Support**: Let your family and friends know how much you appreciate their support and understanding. Positive reinforcement helps strengthen relationships and encourages your loved ones to continue being supportive.
  - Example: *"I really appreciate you checking in with me and being flexible with plans—it makes a big difference and helps me feel included."*
- **Encourage Open Communication**: Let your loved ones know that you're open to questions and happy to talk about your condition if they want to learn more. Encouraging open communication helps dispel misunderstandings and fosters a deeper sense of connection.
  - Example: *"If you ever have questions about my condition or how I'm feeling, don't hesitate to ask. I'm always happy to explain things or let you know what's going on."*

Responding to Well-Intentioned Questions or Comments

During the holidays, you may encounter well-meaning questions or comments from family or friends who are trying to understand your condition but may not know the best way to approach the topic. Responding with patience and understanding helps educate others while maintaining a positive tone.

1. "You Look Fine—Are You Sure You're Not Feeling Well?"

This comment can be frustrating because it dismisses the invisible symptoms of hydrocephalus. Respond by explaining that many aspects of the condition are not visible, but that doesn't mean you're not experiencing symptoms.

- **Response**: *"Thank you for saying that. Hydrocephalus is one of those conditions where a lot of the symptoms aren't visible, but I still deal with things like headaches and fatigue. It's something I manage every day, even if it's not always obvious."*

2. "Why Do You Need to Rest? The Party's Just Getting Started!"

If someone questions your need for rest during a holiday event, explain that taking breaks helps you manage your energy levels and prevent symptom flare-ups. Reassure them that taking a break allows you to enjoy the event for longer.

- **Response**: *"I know the party's just getting started, but taking a break helps me manage my energy and prevents me from feeling worse later. I just need a few minutes to recharge, and then I'll be back."*

3. "Can't the Doctors Just Adjust Your Shunt to Fix Everything?"

Some people may assume that a shunt completely "fixes" hydrocephalus, not realizing that it requires ongoing management. Gently explain that while the shunt helps, it doesn't eliminate symptoms entirely.

- **Response**: *"The shunt helps a lot by draining the excess fluid, but it doesn't solve everything. I still have to deal with symptoms, and there's always a chance of complications, so I need to be careful and listen to my body."*

4. "Isn't Hydrocephalus Just a Childhood Condition?"

Hydrocephalus can affect people of all ages, and it's important to clarify that it's a lifelong condition. Use this as an opportunity to educate others about the nature of hydrocephalus.

- **Response**: *"Hydrocephalus can affect people at any age. I've had it for a while, and it's something I'll manage throughout my life. It's not something that goes away, but I've learned how to live with it and take care of myself."*

Conclusion

Explaining hydrocephalus to family and friends can be challenging, but with clear communication and patience, you can foster understanding and create a supportive environment during the holiday season. By providing simple explanations, sharing how the condition affects you personally, and being honest about your needs, you can help your loved ones understand what you're going through and how they can offer support.

Ultimately, the goal of these conversations is to build stronger relationships based on empathy, respect, and mutual understanding. When your family and friends understand your condition, they're better equipped to support you, helping to ensure that the holiday season is both enjoyable and inclusive for everyone involved.

Chapter 31: Emergency Care During the Holidays
Preparing for Medical Emergencies When Regular Care Is Harder to Access

The holiday season often brings with it a unique set of challenges when it comes to accessing regular healthcare services. Many clinics and doctor's offices have reduced hours or are closed altogether during this time, and increased travel, busy schedules, and social commitments can make it difficult to seek medical attention promptly. For individuals with hydrocephalus, the potential for shunt malfunctions, infections, or sudden health issues means that being prepared for medical emergencies is essential.

In this chapter, we'll explore how to prepare for potential medical emergencies during the holidays, including steps you can take to manage your health, gather necessary medical information, and ensure that you're able to access emergency care if needed. By having a solid plan in place, you can protect your health and avoid unnecessary complications during this busy time of year.

Why Medical Emergencies Are More Complicated During the Holidays

During the holiday season, accessing healthcare can be more complicated for several reasons. Many healthcare providers have reduced hours, and emergency rooms may be busier than usual due to an increase in accidents, injuries, and illnesses associated with holiday activities. If you're traveling, you may find yourself far from your regular healthcare team, making it more difficult to get the care you need from providers who are familiar with your condition.

For individuals with hydrocephalus, these challenges are particularly important to consider because shunt malfunctions or other complications require prompt attention. Delays in treatment can lead to serious health risks, so being prepared in advance is crucial.

Key Challenges During the Holidays:

1. **Limited Access to Regular Healthcare Providers**: Many healthcare offices have reduced hours or close for extended periods during the holidays, making it harder to reach your regular doctor or specialist for non-urgent needs or advice.

2. **Increased Demand for Emergency Care**: Hospitals and emergency rooms may be busier than usual due to seasonal illnesses, accidents, and holiday-related injuries, leading to longer wait times and higher demand for resources.

3. **Travel and Being Away from Your Usual Care Team**: If you're traveling for the holidays, you may be far from your regular healthcare providers and may need to rely on unfamiliar hospitals or clinics for emergency care.

4. **Complications from Disrupted Routines**: The holiday season often disrupts daily routines, which can affect medication schedules, hydration, sleep, and other aspects of your health that are important for managing hydrocephalus.

Steps for Preparing for Medical Emergencies During the Holidays

Being prepared for a medical emergency doesn't mean expecting the worst—it means having a plan in place so that you can act quickly and confidently if a situation arises. The following steps will help you prepare for potential emergencies, ensuring that you can access care promptly and avoid unnecessary complications.

1. Keep Important Medical Information on Hand

One of the most important steps in preparing for a medical emergency is ensuring that you have easy access to key medical information that healthcare providers will need in case of an emergency. This is especially critical if you're traveling or attending events far from home.

- **Create a Medical Information Packet**: Prepare a packet or folder with all of your essential medical information, including details about your hydrocephalus, your shunt, and any other relevant health conditions. Include the following information:
    ◦ A summary of your medical history
    ◦ Information about your shunt, including the type, manufacturer, valve settings, and date of implantation
    ◦ A list of medications you're taking, along with dosages and timing
    ◦ Any known allergies or drug sensitivities
    ◦ Contact information for your primary care doctor, neurologist, or neurosurgeon
    ◦ Emergency contacts, including family members or friends
- **Carry a Shunt Alert Card**: If you have a shunt, carry a shunt alert card that provides critical information about your device. This card is often provided by your neurosurgeon or the shunt manufacturer and contains important details that emergency room doctors will need to know.
- **Make Copies of Your Information**: Keep copies of your medical information in multiple places—such as in your wallet, phone, and luggage—so that it's accessible whether you're at home or traveling. If possible, provide a copy to a trusted family member or friend who may accompany you to medical appointments.

2. Identify Nearby Emergency Medical Facilities

If you're traveling for the holidays or spending time away from home, it's important to identify nearby emergency medical facilities in advance. This ensures that if a medical issue arises, you know where to go for care without wasting time searching for the nearest hospital.

- **Research Hospitals in the Area**: Before traveling, research hospitals or medical centers near your destination that are equipped to handle neurological emergencies, such as shunt malfunctions. Look for hospitals with neurosurgery departments, as these facilities are more likely to have the expertise needed to manage hydrocephalus-related issues.
- **Save Contact Information for Emergency Rooms**: Save the contact information for nearby emergency rooms in your phone or medical packet so that you can call ahead if nec-

essary. Some hospitals allow you to check wait times or contact the ER directly to let them know you're on the way.

- **Familiarize Yourself with Urgent Care Options**: In addition to hospitals, identify nearby urgent care centers that can provide non-emergency medical care. Urgent care centers may be able to handle less severe issues, such as dehydration or minor infections, allowing you to avoid overcrowded emergency rooms.

3. Prepare for Travel with Medical Supplies

Traveling during the holidays can increase the risk of health complications if you don't have access to your regular medical supplies or medications. Preparing in advance ensures that you have everything you need to manage your condition while on the go.

- **Pack Extra Medication**: Make sure you have enough medication to last throughout your trip, plus a few extra days in case of travel delays or unexpected changes. Pack your medications in your carry-on bag if flying, and keep them in a secure place if driving.
- **Bring Hydration and Snacks**: Dehydration can exacerbate symptoms of hydrocephalus, so bring a refillable water bottle and stay hydrated while traveling. Pack healthy snacks, especially if you'll be traveling for long periods or attending events with limited food options.
- **Carry Your Medical Records**: If you're traveling far from home, carry a copy of your medical records and shunt information with you at all times. This is particularly important if you're visiting areas where healthcare providers may not be familiar with your condition.
- **Plan for Accessibility Needs**: If you use mobility aids or have specific accessibility needs, make sure that your travel arrangements and accommodations meet those requirements. This includes ensuring that hotels or event venues are wheelchair-accessible, if necessary.

4. Know the Signs of a Medical Emergency

Recognizing the early signs of a medical emergency is critical for ensuring that you receive prompt care. For individuals with hydrocephalus, shunt malfunctions, infections, or sudden changes in symptoms can quickly become serious if not addressed.

- **Common Symptoms of Shunt Malfunction**: If you experience any of the following symptoms, seek medical attention immediately, as they may indicate a shunt malfunction or blockage:
  - Intense, persistent headaches
  - Nausea and vomiting
  - Drowsiness or difficulty staying awake
  - Visual disturbances, such as blurred or double vision
  - Seizures or loss of consciousness
  - Swelling or tenderness along the shunt tract
- **Signs of Infection**: If you have a shunt, infections are a potential complication that requires immediate medical attention. Symptoms of a shunt infection may include:

- ◦ Fever or chills
- ◦ Redness, warmth, or tenderness near the shunt site
- ◦ Swelling along the shunt path
- ◦ Irritability or confusion
- ◦ Increased fatigue or lethargy
- **Recognizing Dehydration**: Dehydration can exacerbate symptoms of hydrocephalus and lead to headaches, dizziness, and confusion. Common signs of dehydration include dry mouth, dark urine, lightheadedness, and fatigue. If you notice these symptoms, increase your fluid intake and seek medical help if symptoms worsen.

5. Stay Connected with Your Healthcare Providers

Even during the holidays, it's important to stay in touch with your healthcare team, especially if you experience new or worsening symptoms. Many healthcare providers offer ways to stay connected through patient portals, on-call services, or telemedicine options.

- **Use Patient Portals for Non-Urgent Issues**: If you have non-urgent questions or concerns about your health, use your healthcare provider's patient portal to send messages, request prescription refills, or review your medical records. Patient portals are often accessible even when the office is closed.
- **Know How to Reach Your Doctor's On-Call Service**: Most healthcare providers have an on-call service for after-hours emergencies. Make sure you have the contact information for this service so that you can speak to a nurse or doctor if you're experiencing symptoms that require immediate attention but aren't life-threatening.
- **Consider Telemedicine for Follow-Up Care**: If you're unable to see your regular doctor in person due to holiday closures or travel, ask about telemedicine options. Many providers offer virtual visits, which can be a convenient way to consult with your doctor about symptoms, medication adjustments, or other concerns.

6. Create an Emergency Action Plan

Having an emergency action plan in place can help you stay calm and focused in the event of a medical emergency. This plan should outline the steps you'll take if you experience symptoms of a shunt malfunction or other complications during the holidays.

- **Step 1: Recognize the Symptoms**: Be familiar with the signs of a shunt malfunction, infection, or other health issues related to hydrocephalus. If you notice any concerning symptoms, act quickly.
- **Step 2: Contact Your Healthcare Provider**: If symptoms are mild or you're unsure whether you need emergency care, contact your healthcare provider or on-call service for advice. They can help you determine the best course of action.

- **Step 3: Seek Emergency Care**: If symptoms are severe or rapidly worsening, go to the nearest emergency room or call 911. If you're traveling, provide the medical staff with your shunt information and medical records.
- **Step 4: Notify Emergency Contacts**: Let your emergency contacts—such as family members or friends—know what's happening so they can provide support or accompany you to the hospital if necessary.

Tips for Managing Health Emergencies During Social Events

Holiday parties, family gatherings, and other social events are common during this time of year, and medical emergencies can sometimes arise when you're in a social setting. It's important to have a plan for managing health concerns discreetly and seeking help if needed.

- **Communicate with a Trusted Person**: Before attending a social event, let a trusted friend or family member know about your condition and the signs of a medical emergency. This person can help you monitor symptoms and assist if you need to leave the event or seek medical care.
- **Take Breaks as Needed**: If you start to feel unwell during an event, don't hesitate to step away and rest in a quiet area. Taking breaks can help manage symptoms such as headaches or dizziness before they escalate.
- **Know the Location of Emergency Exits**: Familiarize yourself with the layout of the venue, including the location of emergency exits and nearby medical facilities, in case you need to leave quickly.

Conclusion

The holiday season can present unique challenges when it comes to managing medical emergencies, but with careful preparation, you can ensure that you're ready to handle any situation that arises. By keeping important medical information on hand, identifying nearby emergency facilities, staying connected with your healthcare providers, and creating an emergency action plan, you can protect your health and access the care you need—even when regular services are harder to reach.

Ultimately, the key to staying safe during the holidays is preparation. By being proactive and planning for potential emergencies, you can enjoy the holiday season with peace of mind, knowing that you're ready to act quickly and effectively if needed.

Chapter 32: Maintaining Positivity During the Season
Mindset Strategies to Maintain Mental Health and Enjoy the Holidays Despite Challenges

The holiday season is often portrayed as a time of joy, connection, and celebration. However, for individuals with hydrocephalus or other chronic health conditions, the holidays can also bring unique challenges—such as managing symptoms, balancing social obligations with health needs, and dealing with emotional stress. It's important to cultivate a positive mindset that allows you to navigate these challenges while still finding joy and meaning in the holiday season.

This chapter explores mindset strategies to help maintain your mental health, build resilience, and embrace the holiday season despite the potential obstacles. By adopting a proactive and compassionate approach to your well-being, you can focus on what matters most and enjoy the holidays with a sense of peace and positivity.

The Importance of Mental Health During the Holidays

The holiday season can be both physically and emotionally demanding. From attending social events and managing health symptoms to navigating family dynamics and holiday expectations, it's easy to feel overwhelmed. For individuals with hydrocephalus, these challenges may be compounded by physical symptoms such as fatigue, headaches, or sensory overload. Maintaining mental health during the holidays requires a balance of self-care, positive thinking, and realistic expectations.

Fostering a positive mindset doesn't mean ignoring the difficulties you face—it means finding ways to manage stress, practice gratitude, and focus on what brings you joy. The goal is to maintain emotional resilience, even in the face of challenges, so that you can experience the holiday season in a way that supports your well-being.

Common Emotional Challenges During the Holidays

Many individuals face emotional challenges during the holidays, and it's important to acknowledge these feelings rather than suppress them. Recognizing the emotional difficulties that can arise allows you to address them in a healthy and proactive way.

1. Social Pressure and Expectations

The holidays often come with high expectations around socializing, gift-giving, and participating in traditions. You may feel pressure to meet these expectations, even if doing so strains your physical or emotional well-being. This pressure can lead to feelings of guilt, frustration, or inadequacy if you're unable to participate in every aspect of the season.

2. Loneliness or Isolation

While the holidays are a time for connection, they can also evoke feelings of loneliness or isolation, especially if you're dealing with health issues that limit your ability to engage fully with others. You may feel left out of certain activities or overwhelmed by the energy and excitement of holiday gatherings.

3. Stress and Overwhelm

The busy pace of the holiday season can lead to stress, especially when you're juggling health management with holiday preparations. Trying to balance medical appointments, travel, shopping, and social commitments can create a sense of overwhelm, making it harder to enjoy the festivities.

4. Health Anxiety

For individuals with hydrocephalus or other chronic conditions, there may be anxiety around managing symptoms during holiday events. You might worry about experiencing a shunt malfunction, fatigue, or other health complications that could disrupt your plans or lead to an emergency.

Mindset Strategies to Maintain Positivity

Maintaining a positive mindset during the holidays involves cultivating self-awareness, setting realistic expectations, and focusing on what truly matters. The following mindset strategies will help you manage stress, protect your mental health, and find joy in the holiday season, even when challenges arise.

1. Practice Gratitude Daily

Gratitude is a powerful tool for shifting your focus from what's difficult to what's meaningful and positive in your life. By intentionally practicing gratitude, you can cultivate a more positive outlook, even in the face of health challenges or holiday stress.

- **Start a Gratitude Journal**: Each day, write down three things you're grateful for. These can be simple things, such as a kind gesture from a friend, a peaceful moment, or a favorite holiday tradition. Focusing on what's going well helps reframe your perspective and promotes emotional resilience.
- **Express Gratitude to Others**: Take time to express your appreciation to family members, friends, or caregivers who support you during the holiday season. Sharing your gratitude not only strengthens relationships but also reinforces positive emotions.
    - Example: *"I really appreciate your understanding when I needed to leave the party early. It means a lot to me that you support my health needs."*
- **Focus on Small Joys**: During the holiday season, take time to notice and appreciate the small moments of joy. Whether it's sipping a warm drink, enjoying a holiday movie, or spending quiet time with loved ones, recognizing these small pleasures can help you stay grounded and positive.

2. Set Realistic Expectations

The holidays are often portrayed as a time of perfection, where everything is joyful and problem-free. However, it's important to set realistic expectations about what you can do and how the season will unfold. Recognizing your limitations and adjusting your expectations accordingly helps prevent disappointment and frustration.

- **Accept That It's Okay to Say No**: You don't have to participate in every event or meet every holiday expectation. It's okay to say no to invitations or requests if doing so would strain your energy or health. Setting boundaries protects your well-being and allows you to focus on the activities that matter most to you.
    - Example: *"I would love to join you for dinner, but I'll need to leave early to rest. I want to make sure I take care of myself so I can enjoy the rest of the holidays."*

- **Simplify Holiday Plans**: If the holidays feel overwhelming, simplify your plans. Focus on one or two meaningful traditions instead of trying to do everything. For example, you might choose to attend only one or two holiday gatherings or limit your shopping list to a few special gifts.
    - Example: *"This year, I'm focusing on small, meaningful gatherings instead of trying to attend every event. That way, I can enjoy quality time with family without feeling rushed."*
- **Let Go of Perfection**: Perfectionism can increase stress and make it harder to enjoy the season. Let go of the need for everything to be "perfect" and embrace the idea that it's okay for things to be imperfect. Whether it's a small gathering, a simple meal, or a modest gift exchange, the true meaning of the holidays comes from connection and love, not from perfection.

3. Focus on What You Can Control

During the holidays, there are many factors outside of your control—such as other people's expectations, holiday schedules, or even your own health symptoms. Focusing on what you can control helps you manage stress and avoid feeling overwhelmed by the things you can't change.

- **Prioritize Self-Care**: You can't control every aspect of the holiday season, but you can control how you take care of yourself. Prioritize self-care practices that help you feel balanced and energized, such as getting enough sleep, staying hydrated, eating nutritious meals, and taking breaks when needed.
    - Example: *"I can't control how busy the holidays are, but I can control how I take care of myself. I'll make sure to schedule rest breaks and stay mindful of my energy levels."*
- **Create a Flexible Plan**: While it's helpful to have a holiday plan, remain flexible and adaptable. If unexpected challenges arise, such as changes in your health or travel plans, adjust your schedule without guilt. Flexibility allows you to stay focused on what's important without becoming stressed by last-minute changes.
    - Example: *"If I start to feel fatigued during the holiday dinner, I'll take a break and return when I'm feeling better. It's all about listening to my body."*
- **Manage Your Time Wisely**: You can control how you spend your time, so focus on activities that bring you joy and avoid overcommitting. Managing your time wisely helps reduce stress and ensures that you have enough energy to participate in the events that matter most.

4. Practice Mindfulness and Grounding Techniques

Mindfulness involves staying present in the moment and fully experiencing whatever you're doing without judgment. Practicing mindfulness and grounding techniques can help you manage stress, anxiety, and overwhelm during the holiday season.

- **Use Deep Breathing**: When you start to feel stressed or overwhelmed, take a moment to practice deep breathing. Inhale slowly for a count of four, hold for a count of four, and exhale slowly for a count of four. This technique helps calm your nervous system and bring your focus back to the present moment.

  ◦ Example: *"Whenever I feel overwhelmed at holiday gatherings, I step away for a few minutes to practice deep breathing. It helps me reset and return to the event feeling more grounded."*

- **Engage in Grounding Exercises**: Grounding exercises help bring your attention back to the present when your mind starts to race or you feel anxious. A simple grounding exercise is to focus on your five senses—notice what you can see, hear, smell, touch, and taste in the moment. This practice helps reduce stress and anchors you in the here and now.

  ◦ Example: *"When I feel stressed, I focus on the sights, sounds, and smells around me—like the twinkling lights, the sound of music, and the smell of holiday cookies. It helps me stay present and enjoy the moment."*

- **Embrace a Relaxation Routine**: Incorporate relaxation techniques such as meditation, yoga, or progressive muscle relaxation into your daily routine. These practices help reduce stress, promote relaxation, and improve your overall mood during the holidays.

5. Cultivate Connection and Ask for Support

The holidays are a time for connection, and cultivating meaningful relationships can help you stay positive and supported throughout the season. Whether you're spending time with family, friends, or online communities, building a support network allows you to share both the joys and challenges of the holidays.

- **Reach Out to Loved Ones**: If you're feeling lonely or overwhelmed, reach out to family members or friends for emotional support. Talking to someone who understands your challenges can provide comfort and perspective.

  ◦ Example: *"I've been feeling a bit anxious about managing my health during the holidays. Can we talk for a bit? I'd love to get your advice."*

- **Join a Support Group**: If you don't have a local support system, consider joining an online support group for individuals with hydrocephalus or chronic illness. These groups provide a safe space to connect with others who understand your experiences and can offer encouragement.

  ◦ Example: *"Connecting with others in my support group has been a great way to share tips for managing the holidays with hydrocephalus. It's helpful to know I'm not alone in navigating these challenges."*

- **Ask for Help When Needed**: Don't hesitate to ask for help with holiday tasks, such as shopping, cooking, or decorating. Allowing others to support you not only eases your burden but also strengthens your relationships.

  ◦ Example: *"Would you mind helping me with the holiday shopping this year? It's been a bit overwhelming, and I could use an extra hand."*

6. Celebrate Progress, Not Perfection

The holidays are a time for reflection and celebration, but it's important to celebrate progress rather than striving for perfection. Acknowledge the efforts you've made to take care of yourself, manage your health, and participate in the holiday season, even if things don't go exactly as planned.

- **Recognize Small Wins**: Celebrate the small victories, such as attending a holiday event, practicing self-care, or setting healthy boundaries. Each step you take toward maintaining your well-being is worth acknowledging.
  - Example: *"I'm proud of myself for taking breaks during the family gathering. It helped me stay energized and enjoy the time I spent with everyone."*
- **Be Kind to Yourself**: Practice self-compassion and avoid being overly critical of yourself. If something doesn't go as planned, remind yourself that it's okay and that you're doing your best. Treat yourself with the same kindness and understanding that you would offer to a friend.
  - Example: *"It's okay that I had to leave the party early. I listened to my body, and that's the most important thing. I'll have other opportunities to celebrate."*
- **Focus on What Truly Matters**: At the end of the day, the holiday season is about connection, love, and gratitude. By focusing on what truly matters—such as spending time with loved ones, practicing gratitude, and taking care of your health—you can experience the holiday season in a meaningful and fulfilling way.

Conclusion

Maintaining a positive mindset during the holiday season is essential for protecting your mental health and enjoying the festivities, even when challenges arise. By practicing gratitude, setting realistic expectations, focusing on what you can control, and cultivating meaningful connections, you can navigate the season with a sense of peace and resilience.

Ultimately, the holidays are a time to celebrate progress, not perfection. By embracing self-care, asking for support, and finding joy in the small moments, you can create a holiday experience that is both joyful and sustainable, allowing you to enjoy the season while prioritizing your well-being.

Chapter 33: Creating Your Own Hydrocephalus Holiday Survival Plan
Developing a Personalized Plan that Addresses Your Specific Needs for the Holiday Season

The holiday season, while filled with joy and celebration, can also be challenging for individuals managing hydrocephalus. From navigating busy social schedules to managing physical symptoms and addressing emotional stress, it's essential to have a clear strategy to safeguard your health and well-being. Creating a personalized holiday survival plan is a proactive approach to ensure you can enjoy the festive season without becoming overwhelmed or risking your health.

In this chapter, we'll guide you through developing a comprehensive, individualized holiday survival plan that addresses your specific needs. This plan will include practical strategies for managing your health, conserving energy, preparing for social gatherings, and maintaining emotional balance during the holidays. By preparing ahead of time, you can approach the holiday season with confidence and peace of mind.

Why You Need a Holiday Survival Plan

For individuals with hydrocephalus, the holidays come with unique challenges. The increased activity, changes in routine, sensory overload, and the physical demands of travel or socializing can all exacerbate symptoms such as headaches, fatigue, and dizziness. Additionally, managing hydrocephalus often requires careful attention to hydration, medication schedules, and rest—factors that can easily be disrupted during the busy holiday season.

A holiday survival plan helps you anticipate potential stressors, establish boundaries, and prioritize self-care. It also ensures that you're prepared for unexpected changes or emergencies. With a well-developed plan, you can fully enjoy the holidays while protecting your health and well-being.

Key Components of a Hydrocephalus Holiday Survival Plan

Your holiday survival plan should be tailored to your individual needs and circumstances. Below are key components to consider as you develop your personalized plan:

1. **Health Management Strategies**
2. **Energy Conservation and Rest**
3. **Social Engagement and Boundaries**
4. **Travel and Mobility**
5. **Emotional and Mental Health Support**
6. **Emergency Preparedness**

1. Health Management Strategies

Managing your health is the cornerstone of your holiday survival plan. This includes staying on top of your medical needs, monitoring symptoms, and ensuring you have the necessary tools to manage your hydrocephalus effectively.

Stay on Top of Medications and Treatments

During the holidays, it's easy to become distracted and forget about medication schedules or treatment routines. However, keeping up with your medications and other treatments is essential for managing symptoms and preventing complications.

- **Set Medication Reminders**: Use a phone app, alarm, or calendar to set reminders for your medication schedule. Whether you're at home, attending an event, or traveling, these reminders help ensure that you don't miss any doses.
- **Prepare a Medication Travel Kit**: If you're traveling, pack a well-organized medication kit that includes extra doses, your prescription information, and a list of your medications with dosages. Keep this kit in an easily accessible place, such as your carry-on bag or a purse.
- **Stick to Your Routine**: Try to maintain your usual health routine as much as possible, even during the holidays. This includes getting enough sleep, eating regular meals, and staying hydrated.

Monitor Your Symptoms Closely

Hydrocephalus symptoms can fluctuate, especially during periods of increased activity or stress. Monitoring your symptoms and recognizing early warning signs is critical for preventing more serious issues.

- **Track Symptoms in a Journal**: Use a journal or health app to track any changes in your symptoms, such as headaches, fatigue, nausea, or dizziness. This helps you recognize patterns and adjust your activities if needed.
- **Know When to Rest**: Pay attention to the physical cues your body gives you. If you start to feel tired, experience a headache, or notice other symptoms, take a break or rest. Don't push through fatigue—it's important to listen to your body.
- **Plan for Symptom Flare-Ups**: Be prepared for occasional symptom flare-ups during the holidays. Have a plan in place for managing them, whether it's resting in a quiet space, taking medication, or adjusting your activities.

2. Energy Conservation and Rest

One of the most important aspects of managing hydrocephalus during the holidays is conserving your energy and ensuring you get enough rest. Overexertion can lead to fatigue and worsen symptoms, so it's crucial to pace yourself.

Schedule Rest Breaks

During busy holiday events or gatherings, it's easy to get caught up in the excitement and overextend yourself. Scheduling regular rest breaks helps you avoid burnout and ensures that you can recharge before continuing with activities.

- **Plan Downtime**: Before the holidays begin, map out your schedule and intentionally plan downtime between events. For example, if you're attending a holiday party, block off time before and after the event to rest.
- **Take Breaks at Social Gatherings**: If you're attending a large family gathering or holiday party, don't hesitate to step away for a short rest when needed. Find a quiet area where you can sit and recharge before rejoining the festivities.
- **Prioritize Sleep**: Getting enough sleep is crucial for managing hydrocephalus symptoms. Stick to a consistent sleep schedule and avoid late nights whenever possible. If an event goes late, plan to leave early to ensure you get enough rest.

Conserve Energy Throughout the Day

Pacing yourself throughout the day helps you conserve energy and prevents overexertion. Focus on balancing periods of activity with periods of rest to maintain your energy levels.

- **Alternate Between Active and Quiet Activities**: Plan a mix of active and quiet activities throughout the day. For example, if you spend the morning shopping or attending an event, dedicate the afternoon to more restful activities, such as watching a holiday movie or reading.
- **Break Tasks into Smaller Steps**: If you're preparing for a holiday event, such as decorating or cooking, break tasks into smaller steps and spread them out over several days. This prevents you from feeling overwhelmed or fatigued from doing everything at once.
- **Ask for Help**: Don't hesitate to ask family or friends for help with holiday preparations, such as decorating, shopping, or preparing meals. Delegating tasks allows you to conserve energy while still enjoying the holiday season.

3. Social Engagement and Boundaries

The holidays often involve social gatherings with family, friends, and coworkers. While socializing can be enjoyable, it can also be physically and emotionally draining for individuals with hydrocephalus. Establishing boundaries and managing social expectations helps ensure that you stay comfortable during these events.

Set Boundaries Around Social Commitments

It's important to set realistic boundaries around social commitments, especially if you're managing fatigue or other hydrocephalus symptoms. This allows you to participate in holiday events without feeling overwhelmed.

- **Prioritize Important Events**: Decide which holiday events are most important to you, and prioritize attending those. Don't feel obligated to attend every gathering or accept every invitation—focus on the events that bring you joy and meaning.
- **Limit Event Duration**: If attending a long event, such as a family dinner or party, set a time limit for how long you'll stay. Communicate this in advance with the host so they understand if you need to leave early to rest.

◦ Example: *"I'd love to come to the holiday dinner, but I may need to leave after a couple of hours to rest. I want to make sure I'm taking care of my health."*

- **Communicate Your Needs to Hosts**: Let hosts know about your health needs in advance so they can accommodate you. This might include providing a quiet space to rest or allowing you to take breaks during the event.

  ◦ Example: *"I sometimes need a quiet space to rest during social gatherings. Is there a room I could use if I need a short break during the party?"*

Balance Social Time with Solitude

While it's important to spend time with loved ones during the holidays, it's equally important to balance social interactions with moments of solitude and quiet. This helps you recharge and avoid feeling overstimulated.

- **Schedule "Me Time"**: Set aside time for yourself each day, even if it's just a few minutes. This could include reading a book, meditating, taking a walk, or practicing mindfulness. Quiet moments of solitude allow you to decompress from social interactions.
- **Find a Quiet Retreat at Events**: If you're at a large or noisy event, identify a quiet room or outdoor space where you can retreat for a few minutes when you need to rest or clear your mind.

4. Travel and Mobility

If you're traveling during the holidays, especially over long distances, it's important to have a plan in place to ensure that your health and mobility needs are met. Traveling can be physically demanding, so being prepared helps reduce stress and protects your well-being.

Prepare for Travel with Hydrocephalus

Traveling can pose unique challenges for individuals with hydrocephalus, especially if it involves long flights, car rides, or changes in altitude. Being prepared helps ensure a smoother and more comfortable journey.

- **Plan for Shunt Safety During Flights**: If you have a shunt, discuss your travel plans with your healthcare provider before flying. Changes in air pressure during flights can sometimes affect intracranial pressure, so it's important to monitor your symptoms closely.
- **Stay Hydrated While Traveling**: Dehydration can worsen hydrocephalus symptoms, so it's important to drink plenty of water while traveling. Bring a refillable water bottle and stay hydrated throughout the journey.
- **Pack a Travel Kit**: Prepare a travel kit with essential items such as medications, shunt records, water, snacks, a neck pillow, and a copy of your medical information. Keep this kit with you during your travels in case of emergencies.

Plan for Mobility and Accessibility

If you have mobility challenges or specific accessibility needs, ensure that your travel plans accommodate those needs.

- **Check Accessibility at Destinations**: If you're staying at a hotel or visiting family, confirm that the accommodations are accessible and meet your needs. This might include ensuring that there are elevators, ramps, or other mobility aids.
- **Arrange for Assistance at Airports**: If you're flying, request mobility assistance from the airline in advance. Many airports offer services such as wheelchair assistance or priority boarding for individuals with health conditions.

5. Emotional and Mental Health Support

The holidays can be an emotional time, and it's important to prioritize your mental and emotional well-being as part of your holiday survival plan. Managing holiday stress, anxiety, or feelings of isolation is just as important as managing your physical health.

Manage Holiday Stress

Holiday stress can stem from a variety of sources, including social obligations, travel, or family dynamics. It's important to develop coping strategies to manage this stress and protect your mental health.

- **Practice Relaxation Techniques**: Incorporate relaxation techniques such as deep breathing, meditation, or progressive muscle relaxation into your daily routine. These practices help calm your mind and reduce holiday stress.
    - Example: *"When I start to feel overwhelmed by holiday plans, I take five minutes to practice deep breathing. It helps me reset and feel more grounded."*
- **Set Realistic Expectations**: Let go of perfectionism and set realistic expectations for the holiday season. Focus on what matters most and don't stress over small details or trying to meet everyone's expectations.
    - Example: *"This year, I'm focusing on meaningful moments rather than trying to make everything perfect. It's okay if things don't go exactly as planned."*

Build a Support Network

Having a support network of family, friends, or online communities can make a significant difference in how you experience the holidays. Don't hesitate to reach out for support when needed.

- **Stay Connected with Loved Ones**: Reach out to family and friends who understand your health challenges and can offer emotional support. Whether it's through phone calls, texts, or in-person visits, staying connected helps combat feelings of isolation.

- **Join a Support Group**: If you're feeling overwhelmed or isolated, consider joining an online support group for individuals with hydrocephalus or chronic illness. These groups provide a safe space to share your experiences and receive encouragement.

6. Emergency Preparedness

Part of your holiday survival plan should include being prepared for medical emergencies. While you hope to avoid any health issues, it's important to have a plan in place in case of a shunt malfunction, infection, or other emergency.

Prepare for Medical Emergencies

Ensure that you have all the necessary information and resources on hand in case of an emergency.

- **Carry Important Medical Information**: Keep a copy of your medical records, shunt information, and emergency contact numbers with you at all times. This is especially important if you're traveling or attending large events.
- **Identify Nearby Medical Facilities**: If you're traveling, research hospitals or medical centers near your destination that are equipped to handle neurological emergencies. Know where to go in case of a shunt malfunction or other health issue.
- **Communicate with Family**: Let a trusted family member or friend know about your health condition and how to respond in case of an emergency. Ensure that they have access to your medical information if needed.

Conclusion

Creating a personalized hydrocephalus holiday survival plan allows you to navigate the holiday season with confidence, comfort, and peace of mind. By managing your health, conserving your energy, setting boundaries, and preparing for travel and emergencies, you can fully enjoy the festivities while protecting your well-being.

Your survival plan empowers you to take control of your holiday experience, ensuring that you can celebrate in a way that is meaningful, manageable, and supportive of your health. By proactively planning and setting realistic expectations, you'll be able to embrace the holiday season while prioritizing your self-care and emotional well-being.

Appendix
Appendix A: Hydrocephalus Resources
A List of Helpful Organizations, Support Groups, and Medical Resources

Navigating life with hydrocephalus can be challenging, but many resources are available to help you manage your condition and connect with others facing similar experiences. From advocacy organizations to online support groups and medical resources, these tools provide valuable information, emotional support, and guidance on living with hydrocephalus.

This appendix provides a comprehensive list of organizations, support groups, and medical resources dedicated to hydrocephalus. Whether you're seeking educational materials, peer support, or expert medical advice, these resources can empower you to make informed decisions about your health and well-being.

1. Hydrocephalus Advocacy and Support Organizations

Several nonprofit organizations focus on raising awareness about hydrocephalus, funding research, and providing support to individuals and families affected by the condition. These organizations offer educational resources, advocacy efforts, and opportunities to connect with others in the hydrocephalus community.

Hydrocephalus Association (HA)

The Hydrocephalus Association is the largest nonprofit organization dedicated to hydrocephalus in the United States. HA provides education, advocacy, and research support to improve the lives of individuals living with hydrocephalus. They offer a wide range of resources, including webinars, local support groups, and national conferences.

- **Website**: www.hydroassoc.org
- **Resources**:
  - Educational resources about hydrocephalus for patients, families, and caregivers.
  - National and local support groups to connect individuals affected by hydrocephalus.
  - Advocacy programs to raise awareness and support research funding.
  - HA CONNECT, a series of educational webinars on living with hydrocephalus.
  - Annual WALK to End Hydrocephalus events that raise awareness and funds for research.

Hydrocephalus Canada

Hydrocephalus Canada serves individuals in Canada living with hydrocephalus and spina bifida. The organization focuses on education, research, and support, offering programs designed to help individuals with hydrocephalus live independently and thrive.

- **Website**: www.hydrocephalus.ca
- **Resources**:
    - Educational programs and webinars on hydrocephalus management and treatment.
    - Support services, including a helpline and online support communities.
    - Advocacy for healthcare policies that support individuals with hydrocephalus.
    - Educational publications, including newsletters and resources for healthcare professionals.

Spina Bifida and Hydrocephalus Association of America (SBHAA)

While focused on both spina bifida and hydrocephalus, SBHAA offers valuable resources and support for individuals affected by hydrocephalus. The organization works to improve the quality of life for those living with these conditions through education, advocacy, and community outreach.

- **Website**: www.spinabifidaassociation.org
- **Resources**:
    - Educational materials and resources for patients, families, and caregivers.
    - Webinars and virtual conferences on topics related to hydrocephalus and spina bifida.
    - Advocacy initiatives to improve healthcare access and support for individuals with hydrocephalus.

2. Medical Resources and Professional Organizations

Medical organizations and professional groups provide up-to-date information on hydrocephalus treatment, research, and healthcare guidelines. These resources are valuable for patients seeking expert guidance on the latest advancements in hydrocephalus care.

National Institute of Neurological Disorders and Stroke (NINDS)

The National Institute of Neurological Disorders and Stroke, part of the U.S. National Institutes of Health (NIH), provides in-depth information on hydrocephalus, including causes, symptoms, treatment options, and research.

- **Website**: www.ninds.nih.gov
- **Resources**:
    - Comprehensive information on the diagnosis and treatment of hydrocephalus.
    - Details on current research studies and clinical trials related to hydrocephalus.

    ◦ Educational materials for patients and healthcare professionals.

Hydrocephalus Clinical Research Network (HCRN)

The Hydrocephalus Clinical Research Network is a group of hospitals and medical institutions dedicated to advancing hydrocephalus research and improving treatment outcomes through collaborative clinical studies.

- **Website**: www.hcrn.org
- **Resources**:
  - ◦ Information on the latest clinical research studies related to hydrocephalus.
  - ◦ Opportunities to participate in clinical trials or research studies.
  - ◦ Educational resources for patients and families seeking cutting-edge treatment options.

American Association of Neurological Surgeons (AANS)

The American Association of Neurological Surgeons offers information about hydrocephalus from a neurosurgical perspective. Their resources include descriptions of surgical options, including shunt placement and endoscopic third ventriculostomy (ETV).

- **Website**: www.aans.org
- **Resources**:
  - ◦ Information on neurosurgical treatments for hydrocephalus.
  - ◦ Guides on the types of shunts and surgical techniques used in hydrocephalus care.
  - ◦ Articles and publications on hydrocephalus from leading neurosurgeons.

Congress of Neurological Surgeons (CNS)

The Congress of Neurological Surgeons provides medical information on hydrocephalus, focusing on surgical treatments and outcomes. Their resources are valuable for individuals seeking detailed insights into the neurosurgical management of hydrocephalus.

- **Website**: www.cns.org
- **Resources**:
  - ◦ Information on hydrocephalus treatment options, including surgical techniques.
  - ◦ Access to neurosurgical articles and case studies.
  - ◦ Details on the latest advancements in neurosurgery for hydrocephalus patients.

3. Online Support Communities and Forums

Online support communities and forums offer a space for individuals with hydrocephalus and their families to share experiences, ask questions, and provide emotional support. These platforms are especially helpful for those seeking advice from others who understand the challenges of living with hydrocephalus.

Inspire Hydrocephalus Community (Hosted by Hydrocephalus Association)

The Hydrocephalus Community on Inspire is an online forum where individuals with hydrocephalus, their families, and caregivers can share experiences, ask questions, and offer support to one another.

- **Website**: www.inspire.com/groups/hydrocephalus-association
- **Resources**:
  - Peer-to-peer support from individuals living with hydrocephalus.
  - Discussions on managing symptoms, treatment options, and everyday challenges.
  - A safe, moderated space to ask questions and share personal stories.

Hydrocephalus Support Groups on Facebook

Facebook hosts several active support groups for individuals with hydrocephalus, offering a space for real-time discussion, shared experiences, and community support. These groups can be found by searching for "hydrocephalus support" on Facebook.

- **Popular Groups**:
  - *Hydrocephalus Support Group* – A large community where individuals and families share advice and support related to hydrocephalus.
  - *Parents of Children with Hydrocephalus* – A group for parents to connect, share experiences, and offer support to one another as they navigate life with a child who has hydrocephalus.

Reddit Hydrocephalus Community

Reddit's hydrocephalus community is an open forum where individuals with hydrocephalus and caregivers can ask questions, share stories, and seek advice from others who have personal experience with the condition.

- **Website**: www.reddit.com/r/Hydrocephalus
- **Resources**:
  - Discussions on living with hydrocephalus, treatment options, and daily challenges.
  - Anonymous, open discussions where individuals can seek advice or share their experiences.

○ A global community of individuals who understand the unique challenges of hydrocephalus.

4. Educational Resources for Patients and Caregivers

These resources provide in-depth educational materials on hydrocephalus, covering everything from diagnosis and treatment to daily management strategies. They are helpful for individuals seeking to better understand their condition and for caregivers who want to provide informed support.

MedlinePlus (National Library of Medicine)

MedlinePlus, a service of the National Library of Medicine, provides comprehensive information on hydrocephalus, including causes, symptoms, treatments, and medical research. Their resources are written in patient-friendly language and are designed to help individuals make informed decisions about their health.

- **Website**: medlineplus.gov/hydrocephalus
- **Resources**:
    - Detailed explanations of hydrocephalus, including treatment options and potential complications.
    - Links to medical research, clinical trials, and expert articles on hydrocephalus.
    - A medical encyclopedia and resources for understanding related neurological conditions.

Mayo Clinic

Mayo Clinic offers educational resources on hydrocephalus, including descriptions of symptoms, treatment options, and diagnostic procedures. Their materials are written by medical professionals and provide a comprehensive overview of the condition.

- **Website**: www.mayoclinic.org/diseases-conditions/hydrocephalus
- **Resources**:
    - Information on the causes, symptoms, and treatments for hydrocephalus.
    - Patient-friendly descriptions of surgical options, including shunts and ETV.
    - Guidelines for managing hydrocephalus in daily life.

5. Resources for Children and Parents

Children with hydrocephalus and their families often face unique challenges, from managing school accommodations to navigating social interactions. The following resources provide valuable information and support for parents and caregivers of children with hydrocephalus.

Pediatric Hydrocephalus Foundation (PHF)

The Pediatric Hydrocephalus Foundation focuses on raising awareness and funding research for pediatric hydrocephalus. They provide educational resources for families and organize events to support children living with hydrocephalus.

- **Website**: www.hydrocephaluskids.org
- **Resources**:
    - Support groups for parents of children with hydrocephalus.
    - Educational materials on managing hydrocephalus in children, including treatment options and school accommodations.
    - Advocacy efforts to promote pediatric hydrocephalus research and awareness.

The Hydrocephalus Association's Parents and Caregivers Support Network

The Hydrocephalus Association offers a dedicated Parents and Caregivers Support Network, providing resources specifically for families navigating life with a child who has hydrocephalus.

- **Website**: www.hydroassoc.org
- **Resources**:
    - A network of support groups and online communities for parents and caregivers.
    - Educational materials focused on managing hydrocephalus in children, including information on developmental milestones, surgeries, and school support.
    - Webinars and resources on navigating life as a parent of a child with hydrocephalus.

Conclusion

Living with hydrocephalus can be challenging, but a wide range of resources is available to provide support, education, and community connections. Whether you're seeking expert medical information, peer support, or tools for managing your condition, the organizations, support groups, and educational resources in this appendix can help you navigate life with hydrocephalus more effectively.

By staying informed, connecting with others who share similar experiences, and accessing the right support, you can take control of your health and improve your quality of life while managing hydrocephalus.

Appendix B: Medical Glossary
Definitions of Medical Terms Related to Hydrocephalus

Hydrocephalus is a complex medical condition, and understanding the terminology associated with its diagnosis, treatment, and management can help patients, caregivers, and families make informed decisions about care. This appendix provides a comprehensive glossary of medical terms related to hydrocephalus, offering clear, detailed definitions to help you navigate medical discussions and literature more confidently.

A

Acquired Hydrocephalus

A type of hydrocephalus that develops after birth due to injury, infection, tumor, hemorrhage, or other medical conditions. It can occur at any age and is distinct from congenital hydrocephalus, which is present at birth.

Anterior Fontanelle

The soft spot on the top of an infant's head where the skull bones have not yet fused. In cases of hydrocephalus, the anterior fontanelle may bulge due to increased intracranial pressure (ICP) from excess cerebrospinal fluid (CSF).

Aqueductal Stenosis

A narrowing of the cerebral aqueduct (the channel that connects the third and fourth ventricles in the brain), which impedes the flow of cerebrospinal fluid (CSF). This can lead to obstructive (non-communicating) hydrocephalus.

Arnold-Chiari Malformation (Chiari Malformation)

A structural defect where part of the cerebellum (the brain area responsible for motor control) extends into the spinal canal. Chiari malformations can obstruct the flow of cerebrospinal fluid, leading to hydrocephalus.

B

Benign External Hydrocephalus

A condition characterized by an excess of cerebrospinal fluid (CSF) in the subarachnoid space (the area between the brain and the skull). It typically occurs in infants and is considered a benign, self-resolving condition that does not require surgical intervention.

Burr Hole

A small hole drilled into the skull during a surgical procedure to access the brain, typically used to relieve pressure or to place a shunt in hydrocephalus patients. Burr holes are also used in certain procedures like ventriculostomy.

C

Cerebrospinal Fluid (CSF)

A clear, colorless fluid produced in the brain's ventricles that surrounds and cushions the brain and spinal cord. CSF provides nutrients, removes waste, and helps regulate intracranial pressure. In hydrocephalus, the abnormal buildup of CSF causes increased pressure on the brain.

Choroid Plexus

A structure in the brain's ventricles responsible for producing cerebrospinal fluid (CSF). Overproduction of CSF by the choroid plexus can contribute to hydrocephalus in rare cases.

Cognitive Impairment

Difficulty with cognitive functions such as memory, attention, problem-solving, and decision-making. In some cases of hydrocephalus, especially untreated or late-diagnosed hydrocephalus, cognitive impairment can occur due to increased pressure on brain tissues.

Communicating Hydrocephalus

A form of hydrocephalus where the flow of cerebrospinal fluid (CSF) is blocked after it exits the ventricles but is still able to circulate through the brain's subarachnoid space. The term "communicating" indicates that there is no obstruction between the ventricles, unlike non-communicating (obstructive) hydrocephalus.

Congenital Hydrocephalus

Hydrocephalus that is present at birth, often resulting from genetic abnormalities, infections during pregnancy, or developmental issues such as spina bifida or aqueductal stenosis.

Craniotomy

A surgical procedure where a portion of the skull is temporarily removed to access the brain. This procedure may be used in complex hydrocephalus cases to place a shunt or perform other corrective surgeries.

D

Developmental Delays

Delays in reaching milestones such as walking, talking, or motor skills, often seen in children with untreated hydrocephalus due to the increased pressure on the brain affecting normal development.

Dura Mater

The tough outermost membrane that covers the brain and spinal cord. It is one of the three layers of the meninges and helps protect the central nervous system.

E

Endoscopic Third Ventriculostomy (ETV)

A surgical procedure used to treat obstructive (non-communicating) hydrocephalus. During ETV, a small hole is created in the floor of the third ventricle of the brain to allow cerebrospinal fluid (CSF) to bypass the obstruction and flow freely.

Ependymal Cells

Cells that line the ventricles of the brain and the central canal of the spinal cord. These cells help produce and regulate the flow of cerebrospinal fluid (CSF).

External Ventricular Drain (EVD)

A temporary device used to drain excess cerebrospinal fluid (CSF) from the brain in cases of acute hydrocephalus. The device is typically used in an intensive care setting to relieve pressure and monitor CSF flow while a more permanent solution, such as a shunt, is considered.

F

Fontanelle

A soft, membrane-covered space between the bones of a baby's skull. The fontanelle allows for brain growth during infancy. In hydrocephalus, a bulging fontanelle may indicate increased intracranial pressure.

Foramen of Monro

A small channel that connects the lateral ventricles to the third ventricle in the brain. Blockage of the foramen of Monro can lead to obstructive hydrocephalus by preventing the flow of cerebrospinal fluid (CSF) between ventricles.

G

Gait Abnormalities

Difficulty with walking or maintaining balance, often seen in individuals with normal pressure hydrocephalus (NPH). Gait abnormalities may include unsteady walking, shuffling steps, or difficulty lifting the feet.

H

Hydrocephalus Ex-Vacuo

A condition in which the ventricles of the brain become enlarged due to the loss of brain tissue, often seen in neurodegenerative diseases such as Alzheimer's or after a stroke. The enlargement is not due to an excess of cerebrospinal fluid (CSF), as seen in typical hydrocephalus, but rather a compensatory mechanism for brain atrophy.

Hydrocephalus

A condition characterized by an abnormal accumulation of cerebrospinal fluid (CSF) in the brain's ventricles, leading to increased intracranial pressure. It can be caused by a blockage of CSF flow, overproduction of CSF, or poor absorption of CSF. Hydrocephalus can be congenital or acquired and is often treated with shunt placement or endoscopic third ventriculostomy (ETV).

I

Idiopathic Normal Pressure Hydrocephalus (iNPH)

A type of normal pressure hydrocephalus (NPH) where the cause is unknown (idiopathic). It typically affects older adults and is characterized by symptoms such as gait disturbances, urinary incontinence, and cognitive decline, despite normal cerebrospinal fluid (CSF) pressure levels.

Intracranial Pressure (ICP)

The pressure inside the skull caused by the volume of cerebrospinal fluid (CSF), blood, and brain tissue. Elevated ICP can lead to headaches, nausea, vomiting, and, in severe cases, brain damage. Hydrocephalus is a condition that often results in increased ICP due to the buildup of CSF.

L

Lumbar Puncture (Spinal Tap)

A procedure in which a needle is inserted into the lower spine to collect cerebrospinal fluid (CSF) for diagnostic testing or to relieve pressure in conditions like hydrocephalus. It is commonly used to diagnose infections, bleeding, or elevated pressure in the brain.

M
Magnetic Resonance Imaging (MRI)
A non-invasive imaging technique that uses powerful magnets and radio waves to create detailed images of the brain and spinal cord. MRI is commonly used to diagnose hydrocephalus and monitor the size of the ventricles.

Meninges
The three layers of membranes (dura mater, arachnoid mater, and pia mater) that surround and protect the brain and spinal cord. These layers contain cerebrospinal fluid (CSF), which cushions the central nervous system.

Myelomeningocele (Spina Bifida)
A birth defect in which the spinal cord and surrounding membranes protrude through a gap in the spine. It is the most severe form of spina bifida and often leads to hydrocephalus due to the disruption of cerebrospinal fluid (CSF) flow.

N
Normal Pressure Hydrocephalus (NPH)
A form of hydrocephalus that occurs primarily in older adults. Despite the ventricles being enlarged, cerebrospinal fluid (CSF) pressure remains within normal ranges. Symptoms include difficulty walking, urinary incontinence, and cognitive decline. NPH is often misdiagnosed as Alzheimer's or Parkinson's disease.

Neurosurgeon
A medical doctor who specializes in the diagnosis and surgical treatment of disorders affecting the nervous system, including hydrocephalus. Neurosurgeons perform surgeries such as shunt placement or endoscopic third ventriculostomy (ETV) to treat hydrocephalus.

O
Obstructive Hydrocephalus
A type of hydrocephalus caused by a blockage in the normal flow of cerebrospinal fluid (CSF) within the ventricles. Also known as non-communicating hydrocephalus, it is typically treated with surgery to bypass or remove the obstruction.

Occipital Lobe
The part of the brain located at the back of the skull, responsible for visual processing. Hydrocephalus affecting the occipital lobe may result in visual disturbances, such as blurred vision or difficulty with depth perception.

P
Papilledema
Swelling of the optic disc (the point where the optic nerve enters the eye) due to increased intracranial pressure (ICP). It is a potential complication of hydrocephalus and can lead to vision problems if not treated.

Pediatric Hydrocephalus

Hydrocephalus that occurs in infants or children, either as a congenital condition or acquired after birth. Pediatric hydrocephalus requires careful management to prevent developmental delays, cognitive impairments, or physical complications.

R

Radiologic Shunt Series

A series of X-rays or imaging studies used to evaluate the placement and functioning of a shunt system. This test is often used when shunt malfunction is suspected, as it helps identify blockages or disconnections in the tubing.

S

Shunt

A medical device implanted to divert cerebrospinal fluid (CSF) from the brain's ventricles to another part of the body, such as the abdominal cavity (via a ventriculoperitoneal shunt). Shunts help relieve pressure caused by hydrocephalus by draining excess fluid. Shunt systems consist of a catheter, valve, and tubing.

Shunt Malfunction

When a shunt fails to properly drain cerebrospinal fluid (CSF), leading to symptoms such as headaches, nausea, vomiting, drowsiness, and confusion. Shunt malfunctions may be caused by blockages, infections, or mechanical failures, and typically require medical intervention.

Spina Bifida

A congenital condition in which the spinal cord does not fully close during fetal development, often resulting in hydrocephalus. Spina bifida may lead to mobility issues, cognitive challenges, and other complications depending on the severity of the defect.

T

Third Ventricle

One of the four interconnected ventricles in the brain where cerebrospinal fluid (CSF) is produced and circulated. Obstructions in or near the third ventricle, such as aqueductal stenosis, can lead to hydrocephalus.

V

Ventricles

Cavities in the brain where cerebrospinal fluid (CSF) is produced and circulated. There are four ventricles: two lateral ventricles, the third ventricle, and the fourth ventricle. Enlargement of the ventricles is a key feature of hydrocephalus.

Ventriculitis

An infection or inflammation of the ventricles in the brain, often caused by bacteria or other pathogens. Ventriculitis is a serious complication of hydrocephalus that can occur after shunt surgery or other brain procedures and requires prompt treatment with antibiotics.

Ventriculoperitoneal (VP) Shunt

A common type of shunt used to treat hydrocephalus. It drains excess cerebrospinal fluid (CSF) from the ventricles in the brain to the peritoneal cavity in the abdomen, where the fluid is absorbed by the body. VP shunts are a long-term treatment option for managing hydrocephalus.

Ventriculostomy

A surgical procedure in which an opening is created in one of the brain's ventricles to allow cerebrospinal fluid (CSF) to drain. It can be performed as an alternative to shunt placement in some cases of obstructive hydrocephalus.

Conclusion

This medical glossary provides clear definitions of key terms related to hydrocephalus, helping patients, caregivers, and families better understand the condition and its treatment. By familiarizing yourself with this terminology, you can engage more confidently in conversations with healthcare providers and make more informed decisions about managing hydrocephalus.

Appendix C: Holiday Health Journal
Space for Tracking Symptoms and Stress Levels During the Holiday Season

Managing hydrocephalus during the holidays can be particularly challenging due to increased activities, changes in routine, and the physical and emotional demands of the season. Keeping a health journal can help you monitor symptoms, track stress levels, and stay mindful of how your body responds to the holiday hustle and bustle. By recording these patterns, you'll be able to adjust your activities, prioritize self-care, and proactively manage your health to ensure you enjoy the season as much as possible.

This holiday health journal provides space for tracking daily symptoms, stress levels, energy levels, and emotional well-being. It also includes prompts for reflecting on self-care activities, triggers, and what helps you feel better. Using this journal regularly will help you identify trends, manage symptoms more effectively, and communicate clearly with healthcare providers if needed.

How to Use the Holiday Health Journal

- **Track Symptoms Daily**: Use the journal to track specific symptoms you experience each day, such as headaches, nausea, dizziness, fatigue, or any new or unusual symptoms. By keeping daily records, you'll be able to spot patterns and identify when your symptoms may be worsening.
- **Monitor Stress and Energy Levels**: Keep track of your overall stress and energy levels each day. Knowing how holiday activities affect you physically and emotionally can help you adjust your schedule to prevent overexertion and burnout.
- **Record Self-Care Activities**: Reflect on the self-care practices you engage in to support your health, whether it's resting, meditating, or taking breaks during holiday events. Identify what works best for you in managing symptoms and stress.
- **Identify Triggers and Solutions**: Make note of any specific activities, foods, environments, or social situations that seem to trigger symptoms or elevate your stress levels. By identifying these triggers, you can take steps to avoid or manage them effectively.

The entries are best in a separate journal.

Sample Entry Template

Below is a template you can use for each day in your holiday health journal. You can print out multiple copies of this template or create a digital version to fill out daily.

Date: _______________________________

Day of the Week: _______________________________

Overall Energy Level (circle one):

Very Low | Low | Moderate | High | Very High

Overall Stress Level (circle one):

None | Mild | Moderate | High | Very High

Hydrocephalus Symptoms Today:

- **Headaches**: (None / Mild / Moderate / Severe)
  - Description: _______________________________
- **Nausea**: (None / Mild / Moderate / Severe)
  - Description: _______________________________
- **Dizziness or Lightheadedness**: (None / Mild / Moderate / Severe)
  - Description: _______________________________
- **Fatigue**: (None / Mild / Moderate / Severe)
  - Description: _______________________________
- **Cognitive Difficulty (Memory, Focus, etc.)**: (None / Mild / Moderate / Severe)
  - Description: _______________________________
- **Vision Problems (Blurred Vision, Sensitivity to Light)**: (None / Mild / Moderate / Severe)
  - Description: _______________________________
- **Other Symptoms**: _______________________________

Stress Triggers Today:

(Examples: Social events, travel, family dynamics, crowded spaces, loud environments, holiday tasks, etc.)

Self-Care Activities Today:

(Examples: Taking breaks, resting, meditation, hydration, eating balanced meals, etc.)

How Did I Feel After Self-Care?

(Examples: More relaxed, less fatigued, more energized, headaches reduced, etc.)

Activities or Situations That Triggered Symptoms:

(Examples: Large gatherings, loud music, cold weather, travel, etc.)

What Helped Relieve Symptoms?

(Examples: Resting, staying hydrated, taking medication, using sensory aids, etc.)

Reflection on the Day:

- **What went well today?** ____
- **What could I do differently tomorrow?** ____________________________
- **Additional thoughts or feelings**: ________________________________

Weekly Reflection Pages

At the end of each week, consider using a weekly reflection page to evaluate how the week went overall and to plan for the week ahead. Weekly reflections help you step back and assess the bigger picture, including trends in your symptoms, stress management, and the effectiveness of your self-care practices.

Weekly Reflection: Week of _______________

1. **How were my overall energy levels this week?**
   (Were they generally high, low, or fluctuating? What activities drained or boosted my energy?)
2. **How well did I manage my stress this week?**
   (Did I feel overwhelmed, or was I able to stay calm? What caused the most stress?)
3. **Which self-care activities were most effective in managing symptoms and stress?**
   (What practices made me feel better physically or emotionally?)
4. **Did I experience any specific triggers that worsened my symptoms?**
   (Were there any avoidable triggers that I could manage better in the future?)
5. **What changes can I make next week to improve my well-being?**
   (How can I adjust my schedule, activities, or self-care to reduce symptoms and stress?)
6. **What was the best part of my week?**
   (What brought me joy, relief, or connection during the week?)
7. **Additional notes or reflections:**

Tips for Using the Holiday Health Journal

- **Be Consistent**: Try to use the journal daily or at least several times a week. Consistency will help you notice patterns in your symptoms and stress levels, allowing you to make more informed decisions about your activities and self-care.
- **Stay Honest and Specific**: Be honest about how you're feeling, even if it's not always easy to acknowledge. The more specific you are in tracking your symptoms and stress, the more helpful the journal will be in understanding your health.
- **Use the Journal as a Tool for Communication**: If you're seeing a doctor, neurologist, or therapist, bring your journal to appointments. It can provide a detailed record of how your symptoms fluctuate over time, which can assist in adjusting treatments or medications.

Conclusion

This holiday health journal is designed to help you stay mindful of your symptoms, manage your stress, and track your health throughout the holiday season. By recording your experiences and reflecting on what works best for you, you can create a holiday experience that supports both your physical and emotional well-being.

Keeping a health journal empowers you to take control of your health, make adjustments as needed, and ensure that you enjoy the holidays in a way that is manageable and fulfilling.

<u>Message from the Author:</u>

I hope you enjoyed this book, I love astrology and knew there was not a book such as this out on the shelf. I love metaphysical items as well. Please check out my other books:

-Life of Government Benefits

-My life of Hell

-My life with Hydrocephalus

-Red Sky

-World Domination:Woman's rule

-World Domination:Woman's Rule 2: The War

-Life and Banishment of Apophis: book 1

-The Kidney Friendly Diet

-The Ultimate Hemp Cookbook

-Creating a Dispensary(legally)

-Cleanliness throughout life: the importance of showering from childhood to adulthood.

-Strong Roots: The Risks of Overcoddling children

-Hemp Horoscopes: Cosmic Insights and Earthly Healing

- Celestial Hemp Navigating the Zodiac: Through the Green Cosmos

-Astrological Hemp: Aligning The Stars with Earth's Ancient Herb

-The Astrological Guide to Hemp: Stars, Signs, and Sacred Leaves

-Green Growth: Innovative Marketing Strategies for your Hemp Products and Dispensary

-Cosmic Cannabis

-Astrological Munchies

-Henry The Hemp

-Zodiacal Roots: The Astrological Soul Of Hemp

- **Green Constellations: Intersection of Hemp and Zodiac**

-Hemp in The Houses: An astrological Adventure Through The Cannabis Galaxy

-Galactic Ganja Guide

Heavenly Hemp

Zodiac Leaves

Doctor Who Astrology

Cannastrology

Stellar Satvias and Cosmic Indicas

<u>Celestial Cannabis: A Zodiac Journey</u>

AstroHerbology: The Sky and The Soil: Volume 1

AstroHerbology:Celestial Cannabis:Volume 2

Cosmic Cannabis Cultivation

The Starry Guide to Herbal Harmony: Volume 1

The Starry Guide to Herbal Harmony: Cannabis Universe: Volume 2

Yugioh Astrology: Astrological Guide to Deck, Duels and more

Nightmare Mansion: Echoes of The Abyss
Nightmare Mansion 2: Legacy of Shadows
Nightmare Mansion 3: Shadows of the Forgotten
Nightmare Mansion 4: Echoes of the Damned
The Life and Banishment of Apophis: Book 2
Nightmare Mansion: Halls of Despair
<u>Healing with Herb: Cannabis and Hydrocephalus</u>
<u>Planetary Pot: Aligning with Astrological Herbs: Volume 1</u>
Fast Track to Freedom: 30 Days to Financial Independence Using AI, Assets, and Agile Hustles
<u>Cosmic Hemp Pathways</u>
How to Become Financially Free in 30 Days: 10,000 Paths to Prosperity
Zodiacal Herbage: Astrological Insights: Volume 1
Nightmare Mansion: Whispers in the Walls
The Daleks Invade Atlantis
Henry the hemp and Hydrocephalus

10X The Kidney Friendly Diet
Cannabis Universe: Adult coloring book
Hemp Astrology: The Healing Power of the Stars
Zodiacal Herbage: Astrological Insights: Cannabis Universe: Volume 2
<u>Planetary Pot: Aligning with Astrological Herbs: Cannabis Universes: Volume 2</u>
Doctor Who Meets the Replicators and SG-1: The Ultimate Battle for Survival
Nightmare Mansion: Curse of the Blood Moon
<u>The Celestial Stoner: A Guide to the Zodiac</u>
Cosmic Pleasures: Sex Toy Astrology for Every Sign
Hydrocephalus Astrology: Navigating the Stars and Healing Waters
Lapis and the Mischievous Chocolate Bar

Celestial Positions: Sexual Astrology for Every Sign
Apophis's Shadow Work Journal: **:** A Journey of Self-Discovery and Healing
Kinky Cosmos: Sexual Kink Astrology for Every Sign
Digital Cosmos: The Astrological Digimon Compendium
Stellar Seeds: The Cosmic Guide to Growing with Astrology
Apophis's Daily Gratitude Journal

Cat Astrology: Feline Mysteries of the Cosmos
The Cosmic Kama Sutra: An Astrological Guide to Sexual Positions
Unleash Your Potential: A Guided Journal Powered by AI Insights
Whispers of the Enchanted Grove

Cosmic Pleasures: An Astrological Guide to Sexual Kinks

369, 12 Manifestation Journal

Whisper of the nocturne journal(blank journal for writing or drawing)

The Boogey Book

Locked In Reflection: A Chastity Journey Through Locktober

Generating Wealth Quickly:

How to Generate $100,000 in 24 Hours

Star Magic: Harness the Power of the Universe

The Flatulence Chronicles: A Fart Journal for Self-Discovery

The Doctor and The Death Moth

Seize the Day: A Personal Seizure Tracking Journal

The Ultimate Boogeyman Safari: A Journey into the Boogie World and Beyond

Whispers of Samhain: 1,000 Spells of Love, Luck, and Lunar Magic: Samhain Spell Book

Apophis's guides:

Witch's Spellbook Crafting Guide for Halloween

Frost & Flame: The Enchanted Yule Grimoire of 1000 Winter Spells

The Ultimate Boogey Goo Guide & Spooky Activities for Halloween Fun

Harmony of the Scales: A Libra's Spellcraft for Balance and Beauty

The Enchanted Advent: 36 Days of Christmas Wonders

Nightmare Mansion: The Labyrinth of Screams

Harvest of Enchantment: 1,000 Spells of Gratitude, Love, and Fortune for Thanksgiving

The Boogey Chronicles: A Journal of Nightly Encounters and Shadowy Secrets

The 12 Days of Financial Freedom: A Step-by-Step Christmas Countdown to Transform Your Finances

Sigil of the Eternal Spiral Blank Journal

A Christmas Feast: Timeless Recipes for Every Meal

Holiday Stress-Free Solutions: A Survival Guide to Thriving During the Festive Season

Yu-Gi-Oh! Holiday Gifting Mastery: The Ultimate Guide for Fans and Newcomers Alike

If you want solar for your home go here: https://www.harborsolar.live/apophisenterprises/

Get Some Tarot cards: https://www.makeplayingcards.com/sell/apophis-occult-shop

Get some shirts: https://www.bonfire.com/store/apophis-shirt-emporium/

<u>**Instagrams:**</u>
@apophis_enterprises,
@apophisbookemporium,
@apophisscardshop
Twitter: @apophisenterpr1
Tiktok:@apophisenterprise
Youtube: @sg1fan23477, @FiresideRetreatKingdom
Hive: @sg1fan23477

Podcast: Apophis Chat Zone: https://open.spotify.com/show/5zXbr-CLEV2xzCp8ybrfHsk?si=fb4d4fdbdce44dec

Newsletter: https://apophiss-newsletter-27c897.beehiiv.com/

Get printable holiday budget planners: apophisenterprisesllc.org/Apophis-emporium-shop /ols/products/holiday-budgeting-packageprintable

www.ingramcontent.com/pod-product-compliance
Lightning Source LLC
Chambersburg PA
CBHW081911120726
47996CB00010B/3289